Life can only be understood backwards but m
Soren Kierkegaard (1813-1855)

Foreword

When my body talks, it shouts. It shouted me into immovable silence on the day I woke up feeling dead.

This got my attention, all right.

Never before did I have reason to imagine this possibility; what it would be like to wake up one morning and find that I could not move – not my arms, not my legs, not my trunk... only but my head could I move... slowly. It took considerable time before I came to fully realize this – and my response remained stuck in my throat. Such is not a scenario one contemplates – why ever would you?

I felt bewildered, betwixt and between... could not fathom how to explain to the person who came to wake me, that I could not move. I think, if I recall correctly, that I only said that I was too sick to get up.

No, I did not have flu. Yes, I had a headache. No, it was not from alcohol. "But what then, is the problem?" The girl wanted to know from me. I did not know - and could not - explain. And my brain was so fuzzy I did not compute the practical implications – not then, and not for months to come!

I was in Italy in Ruvo di Puglia, touring with a group of Christians and I was the one who had to get up first in the morning to ready the breakfast. And on this particular morning, for once n my life, I could not and did not get up.

Well there I was, left to my own devices as the group went on their day's activities. I did not blame them for leaving me there alone. What could anyone have done to change it anyway? That day I had a cup of tea. Only in the evening did I have something to eat.

Three days in this situation. The group leader did send someone to ask me whether I wanted to be taken to a doctor. My answer was simple: it would be a waste. How am I to explain to an Italian doctor something I could not even explain to my friends in my own language?

Having had months of experience in living in a country where almost no-one could understand English, I knew the need to make do with lots of expansive hand and arm-waving gestures… at that time I was of course not able to use these non-verbal clues! Deep down I also already had within me the realization that the symptom picture presented an inexplicable problem. My brain was too foggy to be able to try and form an explanation anyway.

The group shipped me off to a friend of mine in Rome when they left Puglia. There I lay in bed for 13 days before I managed to get up for more than an hour a day. Already this early in the illness I could sense the lack of understanding of people faced with a sick person whose illness they could not put in some box or other in order to be able to decide how to react/treat the sick individual.

The fact that the illness was inexplicable soon showed me that most people would brush it off as "looking for attention" or a figment of my imagination.

When I at last boarded the flight back to Johannesburg this group to the very last member treated me like a leper. They did not look me in the eye, no-one even wanted to know how I was faring, they fell into silence at my slow approach. Oh well, so much for assistance from Christians…

Also this early, I formed the silent opinion that I could not rely on others. Five years, ten, and twenty years later this has time and again proved to be true. A tiny handful of family members and friends stood by me despite their inability to understand.

Those who were with me on that dreadful day in Italy, left without looking back.

The problem with this shouting my body did, was that it drowned out the music of life. When you can only hear the shouting and little or nothing else, it unbalances you. When you are forced into dealing with the shouting, little remains of the pleasurable things in life – you go around and around the little hamster wheel with little or no perspective.

And might I add that going around the hamster wheel refers to my thoughts and the coping with the illness within my own mind, and not to my physical experience, which had me pinned to my bed… I found out that being sick was hard work.

Thus your perspective becomes focused on the little pinprick of space in front of you. The larger picture disappears, and your experience of life shrinks to within inches of your body.

In retrospect, I now know that the battle I was thrust into concerned not only the spiritual, but also the internal battle between being sick and needing to find answers to become well again, and the overwhelming desire to give up and die. Thus I can never say that I looked the illness in the eye and decided to battle it in order to survive. Yet survive I did.

Chapter One

Waking up feeling dead

Feeling dead or alive. This was not something I ever had reason to ponder. Not until I woke up one morning feeling dead. It was not an emotional feeling of being dead, it was a physical one – a numbness that pervaded my entire body - and yet, with the passage of time, emotional deadness crept into my being and took up residence, making me feel more dead than alive.

That bleak winter morning in 1997 as I came awake slowly, I tried to get up. The first thing I noticed was that I could not move my arms. As I did every other morning of my life, I wanted to lift the covers in order to sit up to get out of bed. Stubbornly, my arms refused to budge. As my brain was not at its brightest either, it did not compute this refusal immediately. Vaguely I realized that something was wrong - very wrong.

Then, of course, my legs refused to comply also. It did in fact take me more than half an hour to fully realize that I could not move. That my body was like a useless lump lying in that cold bed, not willing or able to react to my brain's instructions to get moving – to get up and start the day. I could move my head – slowly – from side to side. But that was all.

In that bed I remained for days, in a fog of fatigued forgetfulness. I had no notion of reality, nor did I care. "What is wrong?" was on every person's lips. (In Italian: che sbagliato?). Not knowing how to answer was a problem in itself.

This was but scene 1

Little did I know that this was but scene one of a life-altering disease that held me in its thrall for more than 15 years. Even now, more than 20 years later, my life – and health – has not returned to normal (that is, normal as

I used to know it). I am in a daily battle to hold on to the shreds of normality, trying to gather them around me like a cloak against the winter cold.

The insipient darkness that entered my being that morning became a constant presence in my life. The fight to rid myself of it has been the theme of my days, nights and every moment my brain could find to interrupt my everyday thoughts.

Making adjustments became the overall life practice for me. Every day was lived within the confines of "who knows what next"… and the brazen reality that my body's energy level could not match that of my brain. In fact, a psychologist once told me that I had the highest level of brain energy she had ever come across. Of course, when your brain commands but your body refuses…you get stuck in a place where you are forced to, come hell or high water, adjust on a minute-to-minute basis, scaling down your expectations of yourself as you go along.

Thus started my struggle against the adversity life had decided to throw at me. Little, very little, has come easy to me. What was once a blossoming career was gone. My career path took an irrevocable downward path. In fact, that is putting it mildly. I did not realize it then, but it, too, died that day. For more than 15 years I had not even thought of the word career. Just being alive was all. That and the everyday nitty-gritty details that life demands attention to.

I did not realize it on that cold morning in the south of Italy, but that was the day that I woke up dead inside. The person I was but a mere 12 hours before had died. The intensity with which I had lived my life was replaced with overwhelming physical pain, supplemented by sometimes intense emotional pain, and at other times, emotional numbness, alongside the physical inability to execute physical movements.

Feeling more dead than alive

From there on I have been carrying this feeling of being dead inside of me – inside my cells and inside my battered psyche. Returning to the person I used to be was impossible. That person, even though not a happy-go-lucky one, never had any perception of the physical, emotional and spiritual cost of chronic, incessant physical pain and the drain on emotions that accompanies it.

I never consciously considered what was happening to me on an emotional level. I had a struggle on my hands that required intense focus on just one aspect of life: physical survival. And it all boiled down to getting through just one day at a time. Attaining this psychological state of mind was more than a mere coping mechanism; it was a necessary means of protection. Yet in reality it also meant feeling emotionally dead. And the start of the long, long road to recover the ability to feel alive while being alive physically, albeit in a much-reduced state of health.

Chapter Two

The doctors and hospitals

While still in Italy I shrank from the idea of consulting with a doctor, simply because I had no way of describing my symptoms to someone who could not understand English. I shut the thought right out of my mind, as to the need to attempt this with hand gestures. And remember, my hands were not complying. Therefore I had rather few options.

So after 13 days with my friend in Rome (lying in a bed in the guest room) I rose and, for all intents and purposes, seemed to return to normal (!) From this stage onwards I could already detect rather negative human reaction... disbelief... lack of understanding... although who can blame others for not understanding, if you could not understand it yourself?

The group that traveled back to South Africa with me kept their distance – as if I was a leper. They looked at me and looked away – they could not accept that my slow movements were due to an inability to do things faster. I think perhaps one of them asked me how I was doing. I noted their reactions but could not be bothered. I had to concentrate very hard to do the things they took for granted: carrying my luggage and making sure I boarded the plane.

Back in South Africa I was feeling decidedly under the weather. I was having difficulty motivating myself and picking up speed. Knowing that this was quite unlike the real me, I eventually formulated the idea of joining a gym. But I should mention here that before this wayward thought took hold and sprouted roots in my mind, a doctor had already mentioned the term that was to be my life companion: Myalgic Encephalomyelitis (ME).

Scene Two of the play

Well, off to the gym and a ridiculous "kiddies sized" program (the instructor had never heard the term ME but was hyper-cautious anyway, thank goodness). Well, this was on my birthday late in August… and ironically, following that session in the gym I did not walk again for three and a half months. This I could neither explain nor understand. I did not try to, either. I did not have the emotional or mental resources to question anything right then. In retrospect, a valid scientific explanation came to the fore eventually, but at the time, well… it seemed ridiculous.

"What do you mean… you can't walk?"

"I cannot get my legs to move"

"What do you mean? Get up and put one foot in front of the other" (actually, no-one said that to me but I could hear them thinking it)

"Are you paralyzed then?"

"No, I don't think so. I sometimes do get upright but my legs do not want to move. They are like lifeless lumps and I have to think hard to get them to move."

"What does the doctor say?"

Some two years down the line the doctor who then treated me explained that due to impaired liver function, my liver had been unable to process the lactic acid generated by my muscles while exercising and that it, therefore, remained in my muscles for months, rendering me unable to move. This explanation did not hold any clues as to what followed. It was just a theory that has now been proven.

The latest (2019) research being done in the US under the leadership of The Open Medicine Foundation is showing that metabolic changes take place in the post-exertional phase (after doing exercise). This is the explanation, at long last. Also brain scans showed lactate in the brain… an inflammatory response found in many CFS patients.

Crawling on all fours - I came to know the patterns on the carpet in my cottage from a close-up perspective. Those days when I did manage to get into an upright position, shuffling in a way that made me look like an octogenarian who had suffered a stroke and was learning to walk again, those were the good days.

Sometimes I did see people staring at me when I with immense difficulty managed to get myself to a shop. But most of the time I had to concentrate so hard on myself that I never noticed anything around me… other than the floor. At this time I had yet to learn that I was in a cycle of relapse/recovery which would last many years into the future.

I was like a drunk without having any alcohol – walking into doors, falling down steps, and breaking crockery and glasses – because while reaching out to pick something up, it did not prove to be where my hand thought it was. Very often after grasping something my hand involuntary opened and it fell to the floor.

Friends and family could not understand that I had dropped off the face of the earth. How could I explain to them that lying in my bed, and hearing the phone ring, could result in a twenty-minute effort to get myself to the other side of the bed, to pick up the phone (I should mention this was before cell phones and before automated answering on landlines)? How could I explain that the very sound of the ringing phone hurt my ears so much that I would start crying?

It now sounds implausible, even ridiculous. Nothing that I did try to explain at the time, made sense to anyone. No-one could understand that I did not just "go to the doctor". Well, I had no job when I returned from Italy, and therefore no medical aid. And of course, no income. So – how could I go to a doctor? As I mentioned earlier I did do that once, but of course, I could not return for more appointments. But the pressure was mounting, because people treated me as though I did not want to get better, as if I was enjoying the pain I was in…!

Hi-ho, hi-ho, off to hospital I go

So came the day that I took off to the Johannesburg General Hospital, the state institution regarded all over the world as a top-notch hospital. Not knowing what to expect, I decided that to arrive early would be the best way to handle the visit. Therefore I left my home at around six in the morning, driving like a geriatric and almost fainting behind the steering wheel. At the hospital I joined the already existing queue.

More than six hours later I was still in the queue. No one dared leave his place for he would forfeit his prized position and would have to join the queue at the back on his return. Therefore, without food or water or a pit stop, there I was: feeling dreadful and not being able to think.

By four in the afternoon, after we had been herded into groups and labeled with stickers to show our medical problems, I was still waiting. By then I had decided that being in my bed would be much better for my body. Thus I fought my way to the front desk and told the nurse to remove my file from the pile in front of her. However, a doctor standing nearby refused to let me go and took me by the arm, asking people to get up from chairs clumped around his desk, and made me sit down. His first question was how I managed to get to the hospital. I told him in my car. He was incredulous… my blood pressure was the lowest he had ever seen and my pulse was 48. He could not believe that I was managing to stand upright and suggested that I should under no circumstances be driving. Well, what could I do? I had no other choice so I drove home. Not without difficulty. But I made it.

This doctor too, suspected that I had ME, and said all he could do for me, was give me a Vitamin B12 injection. He did explain that the diagnosis of ME could not be arrived at with blood tests. Therefore doctors would test for every possible other condition to rule them out, before arriving at the ME diagnosis. And then I was referred to the neuro clinic (this doctor knew that it was neurological). On arrival at the clinic with my letter of referral, I was given an appointment three months later.

Back to Bed

And thus, back to bed, no treatment, no answers, no money, and little food. The latter did not matter much as I was asleep for the better part of the day anyway. And the people. Phew. No-one could understand that a doctor was unable to tell you what was wrong with you, and, on the other side of the coin, that you were not getting better. Their incredulity oftentimes irritated me no end.

How frustrating; trying to explain and fielding these endless questions that had no answers from the other person. Dare I say that at some point I was wishing that I could answer "cancer" just to get away from this perpetual, incredulous questioning and lack of comprehension about my condition.

And so three months slipped past, with darkness being my constant companion. In this phase of the illness I slept around 20 hours a day. The infrequent forays outside my home happened perhaps every 12 days or so. Sometimes I stayed inside my little cottage for ten days at a time without venturing outside the door.

And when I eventually had to brace myself for the long road to the hospital again, it was perhaps with a grain of expectation of receiving answers… or help. Little did I know that my ten o'clock appointment was shared by around 200 others. And so, after throwing my patient card into

the box, started another day of waiting. At three in the afternoon, I saw
the doctor. Who, after several questions, filled in a blood test request
form and sent me on my way. No discussions, no nothing. I tried to ask
questions but answers were not forthcoming.

Well, even an enthusiastic vampire would have given up on me after the
first try. Getting blood from my one good vein was a mission. Those who
knew their stuff realized that they should not use a vacuum tube since it
would flatten the vein and lead nowhere. This first test was for Lupus. And
was negative.

And another one down…

Another week later and another day's wait and another visit to the blood
room. Perhaps not surprisingly, when the nurse saw my face, she asked
me to wait for the nurse I had seen the previous time. She was the local
Nurse Dracula who attended the cases which was akin to getting blood
from a stone. We saw each other a few times.

On one occasion, my veins just did not want to comply, and the nurse
boiled water in a kettle which she upended in a basin and told me to hold
both my arms in the water after adding some cold water to her boiling
cauldron – with the hope of coaxing the veins into showing themselves. I
don't remember very well, but I am sure it worked. I do have another very
clear memory of having blood taken from between the knuckles of my
hand… truly painful.

Years later some of the scenes I experienced at this hospital (and later
also at Steve Biko Hospital in Pretoria) still jump out in 3D in my memory
when I least expect it. Sitting at the Neuro Clinic, waiting hour after
listless, hopeless hour, to be called, the dismal group of sad-looking
unfortunates would sit staring into the distance, while here and there
some would turn to their neighbors and try to start up conversations. This
is where your heart breaks for other people's miseries. Heartaches are
cheap and easy when you listen to these accounts of lives lived in poverty,

in illness and misery which does not seem to present with a light at the end of the tunnel.

Staff attitude

On numerous occasions, while sitting in this holding block in the Johannesburg hospital, one of the patients would fall to the floor, just keel over without warning. No signs of a seizure, which would have alerted the others, just falling over. And those of us who were as yet uninitiated would look expectantly at the nurses' station. No response would come. No-one would make a move towards the person lying on the floor. The first to move would be the people sitting next to the unfortunate person, in most cases one would try and help the person on the floor, and another would get up to call the nearest nurse.

I have seen this more than once. The nurse would walk up to the person on the floor, look down from on high, make no effort to even bend down and take his pulse, or check him, and simply instruct the others to leave him there. Faster than what she had made it to the patient on the floor, she would turn on her heels and walk back to the nurses' station. It was left to the people around him to try and make him comfortable, put something under his head, put a jacket over him. As I said, I have seen this happen more than once. Quite regularly, in fact, so much so that I started expecting it to happen. This is what Albert Schweitzer calls the "fellowship of those who bear the mark of pain".. the empathy of one sufferer with another, so markedly absent in the nursing staff.

What galls me even now while thinking about it, is the attitude of the hospital staff. To them, patients seem to be bugs they try to swat out of their way. On another occasion at the Tshwane District Hospital, I spent more than four hours sitting next to a man with a very deep cut in his foot, from which the blood was dripping onto the floor. After more than four hours playing musical chairs, which left a trail of blood on the floor, he was eventually seen to. Imagine, an accident with an angle grinder leaving you with a gaping wound in your foot, and sitting at the hospital for hours receiving no attention, no medication for pain, while your blood makes a mess on the floor, which not one person pays any heed.

I could only imagine what kind of pain he was in, the blood dripping from his foot and the shock... but no one cared. And might I add, I have seen this same disinterested inhuman attitude in nurses in hospitals everywhere, and not just in the state hospital system. Even in 2017 this was universally evident. I cannot help but wonder what happened to humanity in helping others who are in need.

I can no longer put a time frame on these hospital visits, but I saw eight doctors at the Neuro Clinic over many months. Perhaps the most significant was my last visit to the Johannesburg hospital (and perhaps I should point out that I had received no treatment at all, and my symptoms were still raging unabated). Burning pain in my legs, stiff muscles, vertigo, brain fog, joint pain, sore throat... this was but the beginning.

Helpful advice – if not help

I saw a doctor Jensen. He told me he was convinced that I had ME... And went on to say that no doctor in the state hospital knew how to treat me, and no one had the time to try and find out how. He suggested the only course for me was to find a doctor specializing in the disease. "Don't come back here," he said "you are wasting your time".

Maybe it sounds harsh. The truth often does. Yet he was right. And he did me a favor. There is nothing as soul-destroying as visiting a doctor/hospital and finding no answers, getting no help. Actually, there is. It is a doctor who consults you with a bad attitude, looking at you from on high, disputing the things you say, being rude and uncommunicative. And denigrating your illness as if you were nothing but a neurotic Münchhausen case... or hysterical.

In my personal experience I have found few, very few doctors who were prepared to consult with you after two visits in which they could not pinpoint the cause or decide definitively on the diagnosis. These days not so much about helping the sick but about making money out of disease. I think this is more realistic than a cynical summation of what is out there. Making money is more important than alleviating suffering.

The no-income doldrums

Patients with no income and no medical aid sit and wait at state institutions. When their turn comes, they wait some more. The wheels grind slowly because of the sheer weight of numbers of people who need to be seen. Also in the case of operations, patients sometimes spend days occupying a hospital bed prior to being operated on – a needless waste, and of course, back at work sick leave is taken up while lying waiting to be operated on. This is a reality all over the world, I imagine.

I often wonder how money would have changed the course of this illness. If I had had access to the best (any!) treatment, it might not have lingered in my body for more than 15 years. Still, every year when the winter arrives I battle with my leg muscles – the cold at night means my leg muscles bunch up in protest and the next morning they are stiff and sore. I thought an electric blanket would help this problem – just to find that getting into an artificially heated bed gave me bad heart palpitations. Thus a hot water bottle (the old, traditional variety) remains the only answer – other than the doggie with halitosis which snuggles into bed in the early hours and fashions herself around my body.

How many times have I heard this? "Sore legs? You must take magnesium. Have you heard of the wonder magnesium cream? Your pain will disappear". No understanding of the fact that I do not have cramps, but spasms (due to nerve damage, not muscle pain).

I spent years – literally – to get to the answers I needed. Just being told you have ME does not suffice, especially against the backdrop of the uninformed opinions of those in the medical field. What caused it? A viral infection. Which one? Epstein Barr? Coxsackie? Hepatitis? All of these visited me at some point.

Much of what were bandied about were theories supported by some evidence. Yet they were just theories. As to the exact cause, tracing it back seemed impossible. What I discovered was that so many things played a role, infection, endocrine problems, other pre-existing medical problems, the emotional weight of the situation I was in, and stress. (Briefly, I was sent to Italy as a missionary by my church, who abandoned me there with no support and of course, no income). Looking back, I do not need convincing that the circumstances played a major part in developing ME!

I should note here that ME is indeed a syndrome that takes considerable time to diagnose. In order to reach the eventual diagnosis, clinicians would have to rule out every other clinical condition that could be the cause of fatigue including parasite infestation, connective tissue disease, metabolic disease, heavy metal toxicity, hormonal problems, cancer, AIDS, inflammatory disease and neurological disease. I was tested for most of these (even HIV).

Fatigue indeed accompanies almost all diseases, but the fatigue of ME is usually sudden, debilitating and inexplicable... as inexplicable as going to bed with a headache and sore throat and waking up the next day, unable to move. The first diagnostic criteria for ME is fatigue lasting more than six months.

Feeling tired is not fatigue!

ME was known as post-viral fatigue syndrome long before it was given its present-day name, chronic fatigue syndrome (CFS). It was first recognized as long ago as 1681 by the physician Thomas Sydenham – interestingly he noted that it affected psychologically healthy people and noted (that long ago!) that it was neither hysterical nor psychological in origin.... Not too long ago I still heard doctors and laypeople referring to it as hysterical and even a neurologist I asked in a friendly conversation, said he was not sure but would guess it was a psychiatric illness.

Chapter Five

When mainstream medicine fails

Faced with a doctor who, for one reason or another, failed to help, became a common occurrence. It happens to every person at some point in his or her life. But this takes on significance when, visit after visit to a long line of different doctors, fail to turn up a diagnosis or glimmer of treatment that would alleviate the pain and suffering, especially when one is so sick that you cannot work – and therefore do not generate an income.

It would be interesting to know the number of people who fall into this category – which means they are dependent on state medical facilities (in South Africa) unless of course they were medical aid members before falling ill. Then, even medical aid cover is not unlimited and runs out in due course – leaving those people also without help.

As I have mentioned, by the time I had seen eight neurologists (and had visited the Rheumatology and Hepatology clinics) the consensus on the diagnosis had been reached. As had the admittance that they did not know how to treat ME. This dragged out experience is not uncommon. Several disease conditions require multiple visits and investigations prior to the definitive diagnosis. But ME stands in the dock alone, awaiting the sentence of "no known treatment".

Alternative answers – alternative methodologies

Some patients already before reaching this stage turn to the field of alternative or complementary medicine for answers and help. I would venture to say that it happens to most patients eventually. The variety of alternatives is almost endless and the chosen therapy will probably depend on the most important symptoms: as ME patients do not all present the same set of symptoms with the same severity. In my case the muscle spasms in my legs were the overriding problem, alongside fatigue, of course. Other patients I have had contact with, did not have the muscle

pains but rheumatic-type joint pain, abdominal pain, depression —
coupled with our faithful friend fatigue.

Being unable to move, to walk, was evidence enough that something was
seriously wrong with my body… and slowly, after numerous brushes with
doctors and hospitals, I started taking control as well as responsibility for
my debilitating disease; and the management thereof.

According to Scott Peck, the problem of distinguishing what we are and
what we are not responsible for in this life is one of the greatest problems
of human existence.

This is not to say that it was easy, nor was it a one-time realization that
led to a one-time management plan, rather it was a slow process in which
I sometimes took heart when having had a day in which I managed to
overcome the physical limitations and do something I felt proud of. No-
one I contracted with for work in those days, ever knew that it took a
gargantuan effort for me even to walk. Thankfully the work I produced
was of such a standard that I maintained my work contracts on a level
where I earned enough to stay alive.

So, for me, trying physiotherapy was useless, because my muscles had the
consistency of cement. The answer to this took a long time in coming but I
did eventually find out why my large skeletal muscles had gone into this
non-responsive state.

Homeopathy

I have had many homeopathic treatments (even though my church told
me Samuel Hahnemann had been a Satanist and Christians should not use
his methods) and have always found homeopathic interventions
successful. One has to, of course, understand the principles and follow the
treatment as prescribed. Furthermore, expecting the deadening
properties of a pain-killer from a systemic treatment modality that
changes the body on a cellular level over the long term, is the kind of
thinking that sees many scoff at homeopathy.

for) and secondly, I knew already that some supplements like magnesium and calcium were contra-indicated since my body was not able to metabolize them. In fact, magnesium turned me into an acidic blowfish of note.

And then; the food allergies and food/chemical intolerances. People nowadays are more aware that food can be harmful, thanks to becoming more educated on adverse reactions to food and food additive substances. Even so, in restaurants, I have had situations where I ordered a salad without cheese, and then being served the cheese anyway – and when I asked them to bring me a new salad, had to witness the waiter standing at the counter picking the cheese out of the salad with his fingers! On other occasions, when asking for rye bread, and requesting margarine (I am allergic to cow's milk) I have been told that the restaurant only keeps butter, and not margarine. This is absurd! As for wheat-free bread.. let's not even go there.

I still wonder why restaurants in South Africa are not more aware that there are literally thousands of people who are allergic to dairy and also wheat. Why they do not have alternatives on hand as standard practice? Some waiters even laugh when you tell them about being allergic. Many, very many, people do not take it seriously.

Indeed eating in a restaurant is a demanding experience. First I scan the menu and eliminate the obvious. Then, one can get caught on things not mentioned on the menu, like the random dipping in soy sauce… or grilled veggies being smothered in butter before grilling. What seems innocuous to most people, could have dire consequences for me and I have spent hours and money in righting problems arising from eating the wrong food – having to be put on a drip to counter the reaction.

Isolation

Being confined to a bed, crawling around, shuffling when upright, having difficulty stringing words into sentences – is it any wonder that these things all work together to isolate you quite effectively? And years down the line, seeming totally healthy, able and fine, still feeling isolated because your energy level still cannot quite match that of normal people? When they keep going, you meander to your bed knowing that your flat battery needs recharging. A social dampener, that is.

In terms of planning outings, this was always at the top of the list... how long would I have to keep going before I would be able to rest again? In the early days of recovery, just walking was close to impossible. Climbing one flight of stairs needed planning; stops to rest and a considerable amount of time... making others impatient and even annoying them.. since you are rather young you should not be struggling to alight a flight of stairs?

Years of this struggle and being at the receiving end of other people's reactions, knowing they could not possibly know, or understand, nor would they care, makes you retract into your mind and stay there. I have not asked other sick people about this but I am rather certain that they experience the same sense of isolation. This is easy to understand when a person is bed-ridden. But how can one know what another person is experiencing when just the act of going up a flight of stairs, or traversing a shopping center, is a mammoth task kept for a special day... when energies have been saved up and kept aside for this excursion?

But talking about isolation, I have felt this emotion keenly on many levels: physical, emotional and spiritual. I have to admit, not only could other people no longer relate to me, I struggled to relate to them. How could I understand a friend's emotional rollercoaster of being-in-love problems, when my life had been denigrated to the problem of getting up, of moving, of standing, of walking?

Likewise, how could she reach down and find an understanding of my life situation? This is where expectations take a dive too. One's expectations of life - and people - get taken down more than just a few notches – it dives right through the floor. Over time one's emotional reserves increase to a stable level where once again you can relate to others, even if you still feel a sense of isolation.

is living on earth – or, alternatively, total despair and seeing no other choice than giving up. Think of Vincent van Gogh.

Philip Yancey describes the effects of pain as grinding down the soul toward despair and hopelessness. I have also heard of pain drowning out one's faith.

I eventually came to relate to Tantalus – although I could not pin down the wrong I had done to be in this situation. He, after all, knew exactly why he was being punished – I am still trying to figure out why. Like Tantalus, I felt unable to reach for that which I tried to attain every single day of my life, with resultant frustration. In fact, frustration has become my middle name, part of my personality. A part which I try to deny, and cover-up. But it is there all right. And like Tantalus, I can see, I can reach out, but I cannot grasp. There is no rest, no let-up, no peace.

Yet; "There is a force, the mechanism of which we do not fully understand, that seems to operate routinely in most people to protect and encourage their physical health even under the most adverse conditions" said Scott Peck. He said in The Road Less Travelled also "within each and every one of us there are two selves, one sick and one healthy – the life urge and the death urge, if you will".

So – when you fall ill you meet this other self, and from there on the journey starts with "revising your map of reality" as he puts it.

The meaning of death - having a death wish

Most people will probably assume that having a death wish is tantamount to being suicidal. This is not necessarily true. I have fought this fight, wanting, wishing myself dead, but having to stay alive. Against my wishes, I have not been given the grace to die. Nor have I found that all-encompassing *raison d'etre*… the meaning and reason for being alive, in worldly terms. My own self has not rebelled at this. I accept that God has the say over life and death. And even if you find no other reason for being (and staying) alive, that should be enough.

Could it be that reaching into the illness brings spiritual growth? Scott Peck postulated that there is a powerful force outside of human consciousness which nurtures spiritual growth. I can say that I have grown away from where I used to be. Emotionally and spiritually.

Chapter Eight

Getting up after falling down: the early days

Long gone were the limitless days of careening through the day, mindless of my body's needs. Now my body was talking louder than my mind, and I was forced to listen.

Coming to terms with not being able to walk, or move your arms, not being able to lift them to dry your hair, in the early days, was far from easy. However, when everything is in shut-down mode, you do not dwell on the individual things you cannot accomplish. You are down and out, period. There is only one shade of grey in this picture – dark grey. Very dark, fading to black, living towards that tiny little pinprick of improbability where my real self resides; in my brain. That place where life resides without any reason, and where you grope and grapple to find, and release it.

But later on, as you regain some smidgeon of normality, you become aware of the smaller details of which things you can do, and which ones are beyond the scope of things you can do without careful consideration. The things you do every day without thinking are the things we all take for granted. Being able to dry your hair is one example.

Who needs to consciously think about the action required to pick up and hold a hairdryer in position to dry (style) one's hair? Only those people who cannot do so. If you have never had to think about it, count yourself blessed. The thing is, we never do until we find ourselves in a position where we realize just how much we take for granted!

belief of getting through one day at a time. Much like the AA 12-step program, especially in the early days of being dreadfully ill, I considered success to be when I made it through another day. Some days were good – and others made me wish I had fallen off the side of the earth. And in this came the ability to get up one more time, even if the previous day was not a great one, and the day looming ahead was fraught with uncertainty.

This was true right from the start. Gritting one's teeth and biting into the fact that you don't feel like it, that your body does not want to respond, yet you get up and you get going. Does this take guts, do you think? Perhaps.

Considering the alternative as just staying in bed, lying there, not participating in life…once again, I reiterate it was not really a conscious feeling of wanting to be alive or to prove anything, it was just something I did. And, not always because I wanted to.   One might think of this as the magnitude of the mental force at work.

Chapter Ten

Negative emotions

As if being dreadfully ill was not enough, having to cope with the negative feelings that go along with having to rise above the pain, the draining fatigue and the other symptoms like muscle spasms or heart palpitations, on top of this came the bad feelings engendered by others… such as hospital staff, as I mentioned before.

In the beginning, hopelessness would descend as you stand in front of a person who just point blank refuses to listen to you or answer a question. The blank lack of interest would irritate you mildly. Later it would irritate you in a more pronounced way and one day it will have you rise to the heights of anger.

This anger is stirred by the realization that human beings (not just you, but everyone around you) are being treated like animals. They are not given the time of day or treated with any sign of interest (there are exceptions, I should hasten to add – a few,) but they are to be not easily found. Nursing staff complain about patients. All-day long they keep up a song of complaint. Yet they treat the very people they supposedly feel called to help, like some hurdle in their path to a glorious day on the job.

Rising Anger

I have seen others become angry, and within me felt the stirring of anger on their behalf. Later I became angry for my own sake. Still today, I feel my ire rise when thinking of how people are treated in hospitals... people who have no resources and no other recourse – left in the hands of disinterested and in many cases, incompetent, staff.

This is not a plea for sympathy. It is a concern for humanity. From my own perspective, I can say that if you are constantly treated like a non-human or less than a human being, you start feeling less than human. Even doctors in private practice treat patients like this. I have experienced it many times. Some of them do not even bother to do an examination (even specialists, might I add), and send you out of their practice with nothing other than a large bill. Anger? What anger?

Do medical staff receive absolutely no training on how to deal with sick people? Do they have no understanding that the way they speak to people play a role in people's wellness? Or are they so uncaring that it does not matter to them at all?

I have had many ME sufferers contact me and have seen and experienced their anger, as well as my own. In all these years I have found perhaps five medical practitioners that did not scoff, or treat me like a freak show put up for amusement, or with total professional disdain. In these five people only have I found someone prepared to go all the way, to stay on the route to helping someone to recover. One doctor went out of his way, explained, is a lesson in how to think about the illness. The person carrying the suitcase has to make up his mind how to deal with the load to stay balanced.

If he has to go uphill with the suitcase, he may decide to stop every couple of steps and rest, or may well decide to remove some items from the suitcase to make it lighter and easier to cope with. This allegorical depiction applies to all disease conditions, or even crises or stressful situations in life.

Sitting here, contemplating my present car problems, I am trying to imagine it as being the suitcase… and trying to figure out how to shift the load of the stress so that I can regain my balance and face the day with confidence and not have this nagging worry about where (or whether) the car might leave me in the lurch!

Angry at the illness, angry at myself – angry at God

I imagine any person wracked with pain or other symptoms probably become angry at some point. Just consider some of the people you have seen in old age homes! Angry at the pain, the inability to perform certain actions or tasks, angry at life, angry at feeling disabled. By the way, in the UK, ME patients are classified as disabled. And quite frankly, during the first six years or so, I was little more than that. I did not manage seven days out of seven on my feet (even though no-one noticed because, as it is, people only see you when you are on your feet and have absolutely no idea how many hours you spend lying in your bed.)

One very big plus when an illness drags you into oblivion is that you question everything, every word people say, everything you read and everything you have ever believed to be true. From that very first day onward I have never point-blank believed anything again. Not on any level of my life. Cynical? Perhaps. Cautious? Perhaps. But never again will I accept any statement without weighing it, researching it, and praying it.

Hoo boy. What a wringer illness is. Apart from the medical fraternity's apathy and negativity, on the other hand I had my church. A whopper of a charismatic church. Whose members all held firmly to the health doctrine as propounded first by the charismatic pioneers Kenneth Copeland and Kenneth Hagin. The firm belief was that Christians cannot be sick. I have heard every version of every verse and every sentence and every explanation. Some came at me with "you are disobedient and God is punishing you"… others held that I have sin in my life and should confess it and I would be healed.

Others were of the opinion that I was demon-infested and under the control of Satan. And then, when you have been prayed for, and do not immediately jump up and dance around, and they see you weeks later, they are astonished to hear that you have been ill in bed. "But we have prayed for you?" Incredulous response.. after which follows the insinuation that it is somehow your fault that "you have not received your healing" because "God gave it to you when we prayed…"

Condemnation

Thereafter followed, from Christians, not loving help, but condemnation. "You are in unbelief, which is a sin before God. He will heal you if you believe." If I was not so dreadfully ill I would have laughed at some of these antics. One day sitting at a friend's house waiting for someone to pray for me, when the troops gathered round I was ordered to stand up. I answered that I did not have the strength to stand. Then was told that, if I did not have enough faith to stand, how would God heal me? Well, I can but wonder that God would be unable to heal me just because I was sitting down and not standing up?! I could not in subsequent attempts find evidence that God heals only people who have faith – or standing up.

I thus embarked upon an intensive search for answers in the Bible. And found that the so-called healing doctrine had been arrived at in this way: taking the Strong's Concordance and looking up every single verse to do with all the words related to healing. These verses had been thumped into me in the twenty or so years I spent in the Charismatic movement.

Numbness and a burning sensation at the same time? It sounds incongruous. Impossible. As if you are making it up. Yet it was true. I understand fully that there are people who escalate their symptoms to make it more important or struggle to explain what they are experiencing because they cannot pin it down with words, but I have always tried to be clear on this since I understand that doctors can only go on what you tell them.

ME though is like looking for a needle in a haystack – so many symptoms, so many clues and also a number of red herrings. If I hadn't found a doctor specializing in the disease I wonder even now how things would have turned out. This doctor in Johannesburg would look at me and say: "I think you have a low potassium level" and this would be borne out by a blood test. Not many doctors (in fact pathetically few of them) knew where to look for clues.

This is where the word holistic became a reality in my life. ME can not be addressed symptom by symptom, but since it is a syndrome, it has to be seen as immunologic/metabolic/neurologic in essence and treated holistically. Just like 'one swallow does not make a summer' one symptom or even group of symptoms cannot be treated in isolation.

And back to the pain. The deadness in my muscles. The inability to move. Crawling and shuffling when upright. The battle to overcome the refusal of my muscles to do what I needed them to do.

People who have been rendered paralyzed with the possibility of rehabilitation, know what I am talking about. You have to think about every movement. Look at your arm, visualize it doing what it would have been doing without being told: these involuntary movements your body performs millions of times on a subconscious level.

Emotional doldrums

Emotional responses to chronic pain has been studied more in recent years. If only doctors would heed these studies! From the research it is clear that emotions and the cycle of pain are interrelated. Just as emotions may impact physical pain directly, the reverse is also true. Physical pain exerts emotional stress in turn. If you are stressed your muscles tense and pain is the result. And when your muscles are in pain, your emotions will become repressed or depressed.

"Believing that you have control over your life and can continue to function despite the pain or subsequent life changes has been shown to decrease depression." This is according to a research paper: "The emotional impact of the pain experience". (2008)

I lived with this for years. Hopelessness is a pervasive emotion and can drag you down into depression. I most certainly experienced depression in waves or should I say pits. Control.. what do you have control over, other than perhaps the most basic bodily functions... unable to walk, unable to work, unable to look at yourself in the mirror, having lost your self-esteem... lack of control lowers you into depths where others cannot reach.

In fact, chronic pain changes your identity, chipping away at your individuality. How you used to define yourself may be less of an issue than having to redefine yourself as a person with impaired life choices, a changed lifestyle and limited future outlook. In short, being disempowered changes who you are.

And, says the research ..." depending on what roles or characteristics are most valued to an individual, impairment in that area will most affect his identity and make the pain feel more pronounced." For someone like me, who defined myself in terms of the things I could do, the skills I had amassed, being "functionally paralyzed" (my own term) meant my entire self went down the drain.

The invisibility of pain can be isolating, especially in cases when a person's outward appearance remains the same. This was true in my case. I used to think of people not realizing my agony in the early hours (and late) since they could not see a change in my overall appearance, not such as losing my hair or emaciated muscles would have done if I had had cancer.

body is programmed to heal itself, and will do so, with a little help. Norman Cousins discovered this for himself also. Candace Pert pointed to the fact that compassion from a doctor, the patient's awareness that the person is caring and want to help, and, as she pointed out loving touch (such as used in touch therapy and manifested in the laying on of hands favored by faith healers) plays a definitive role in mobilizing the body's own healing processes.

Deepak Chopra points to the fact that no-one raises an eyebrow when receiving a superficial cut on the body which heals by itself, without intervention. The body's action is that of intelligence – which no-one can truly pin down: is it seated in the brain's electrical impulses, neurochemistry, or is it the mind? It is not merely mind over matter either since very few people actively THINK about their body processes that kick in when they have a cut on a finger. Yet, doctors stand amazed at what they refer to as "Spontaneous remission" of cancer… or any other signs that the body has healed itself.

Somewhere along the line medical students seem to lose the desire to help people, which, supposedly, is why they decided to enter the medical profession. And this goes for nurses too. I have seen downright rudeness, refusal to help patients, indifference… the entire spectrum of negative treatment of patients. My aunt, who spent her entire career as a hospital nurse, who was hospitalized recently, sighed resignedly when she described how only one nurse in her more than three-week stay in a private clinic, bothered to treat her humanely.

Hospital woes

No wonder Norman Cousins, who fought his way back from a fatal affliction, said a hospital is no place for a person who is seriously ill. He pointed to the sacrosanct discipline of hospital regimes. A patient who struggles to sleep will be rudely shaken awake at 5 am because hospital rules say it is time for breakfast, even if he had dropped off just an hour before for the first time that night. Might one remember that rest is an integral (if not the most important) part of regaining one's health?

The body gets stopped by illness in a bid to slow it down enough for regeneration to kick in – since we all rush around like mindless minions, taking almost no cognizance of the fact that we are actually abusing our bodies.

I have learned never to underestimate the capacity of the human mind and body to regenerate – even when the prospects seem most wretched.

The question is how many doctors play into the negative... by their words and reactions, they make the patient feel hopeless, feeding into their despair and contributing not to their wellness, but their illness. Patch Adams comes to mind again – he came up against the demi-God doctor who treats the patient without giving a thought to his mind, his thought processes, his being human before being a patient. This has become the norm – even if not normal!

What I find surprising is that Norman Cousins wrote at length about this – *in the early seventies*. And apparently in the US doctors have heeded some of his comments at that time. From everything I have said on this subject, it is clear that in South Africa, we have a long way to go in this respect. When I compare the doctors who qualified earlier with the younger batch, I cannot say that things have improved. Of the three persistent Petes, I have come across one was in her thirties, and two in their fifties. I know another Pete but he is a naturopathic physician who turned his back on traditional Western Medicine.

Cousins points out in his book that he received letters from 3 000 doctors, and said that the letters reflected the view that "one of the main functions of the doctor is to engage to the fullest the patient's own ability to mobilize the forces of mind and body in turning back disease".

If only... if only this could be true. I have had this experience maybe twice. After years of being ill, I now count myself as healthy (note: not "healed") since my body has eventually restored itself. Doctors and medical treatment had very little to do with it. Cousins said those 3 000 doctors have to believe in Kenneth Hagin, or should I believe in the Bible? (The choice is obvious to me).

What you think and **how** you think is based on what/who you believe in. At this point I started rediscovering my Christian beliefs. And the conclusion I eventually reached, and still hold on to, is that one should be really careful with churches and what they preach.

Finding meaning

When you get hit by a drop-down disease, finding meaning in your situation is very far from your conscious mind. Eventually though, you start asking many questions about how, and what the reasons are for your predicament and how to get out of it – as soon as possible. For me, as the months and then the years dragged by, I ceased my search for information on the disease and treatment options that could lead me back to health after some years of trying.

I still read up on ME and the latest research from time to time, but it is not my focus at all. Also the search for treatment (be it naturopathic, homeopathic, alternative, complementary, or whatever) has no meaning for me anymore. I had reached a point after probably five years when this became fruitless. I should add that I had tried some of the options I uncovered, some worked well and others I discarded.

I think my body rallied and healed itself over time. This is what the human body is programmed to do. My psyche still wages war and battles with the thoughts that accompanied becoming a human vegetable. Lack of self-worth is but the basis on which many other self- denigrating thought patterns are built. Unfortunately, the way others treat you perpetuates your own feelings of not being worthy. And this is a circle of negativity that could be termed a self-fulfilling prophecy.

But to find meaning in the midst of these circular patterns of problematical pondering... where do you go?

Frankl said he grasped the meaning of the greatest secret that human thought, poetry, and belief had to impart: The salvation of man is through love and in love.

I am not sure that I understand this fully. I still battle with the meaning of the word love. But he came to this conclusion after explaining how some inmates withstood the rigors of camp life by finding an inner place in their minds to escape to. He equated this with love because he escaped to a place where he thought of his wife and the love he had for her.

Ability to escape

I wonder whether this was really about love, or was it rather about the ability to escape?. After all, we can find places to escape to inside our thoughts without equating it with the love for another human being. Personally, I did not have a person to hang my thoughts on, someone which I could focus, on whose behalf I could hang my dignity in suffering.

My thoughts pretty much focused on asking God what he wanted from me. In fact, what the meaning of the illness was. I never once asked the "why me" question. I did have, and still have, the need to know what it was that falling ill and losing my life as it were, had to teach me. In honesty, I am still searching for an explanation. This process is what Scott Peck termed Spiritual Maturity.

Maybe it is as simple as Nietzsche's point that if it does not kill you it makes you stronger. Maybe. And then again, perhaps some people's destiny is to suffer, as Frankl concluded. He said that if a man finds that it is his destiny to suffer, he will have to accept his suffering as his task. He postulated that such a man's unique opportunity lies in the way in which he bears his burden. That could be it. No heights to scale, no career ladder to climb, and one advantage is that you cannot really fall because you are not very high up!

Initially one does not think about losing – or having lost - your career. You are totally focused on survival. Over time, though, as you go through life being treated by others like a lesser being, spoken down to because you

Having gained a larger than normal amount of medical knowledge (partly due to my job as editor of a medical journal, and partly from studying physiology as part of a herbology course) I am going down this road to athletic participation with not only caution but intelligent planning.

My one ankle gave me cause to consider. My intention remained the same, after having had X-rays done, consulting with a doctor and physiotherapist, I concluded that nothing was really wrong: intelligent shoe choices were called for.

I now wonder whether I had always been this way, taking the analytical approach and giving due consideration to things before taking a leap. And this rather funny incident comes to mind. While working for Liberty Life many years ago, I (like the rest of the staff) was sent on a social style course. This called for five people filling in a confidential questionnaire about you, and this being sent to the USA for number crunching and your profile is identified as a combination of two of four quadrants.

These quadrants identified your overall social style as being driver, expressive, analytical or amiable. Then a two-day workshop took place during which all this was shared. On the second day of the workshop each person was handed his/her profile – straight from overseas.

Well, I opened mine and looked at it. Then I raised my hand and asked to say something. The course facilitator said go ahead, and I saw her smile grow larger with every word coming from my mouth. I listed in point form reasons why I thought the course was a waste of time and money. When I stopped speaking, she asked me to tell everyone what my profile identified my style as being and well, they fell around laughing when I answered "expressive analytical" and she had reason to point out that it was quite accurate since I had just demonstrated it with the way I behaved.

Thus, no, the illness did not make me analytical. Yet, perhaps it is this side of my nature which had me weigh everything – as I am still doing now – and reacting to my physical problems in the way I have. Discarding and disregarding the medical profession and its input on many occasions, albeit not in its entirety, and taking responsibility for how I regained and maintain my health, rests squarely on this part of who I am.

I did not, and never would, rush in and try something, but first I read, analyze and then make decisions based on the information I have. As I have said before, if you turn your back on Western medicine you can land in a quagmire of quackery which will embrace you; and its actors, or proponents, may well try to get you involved in things you should rather stay away from.

I don't go for just anything. I followed a course in herbology and firmly believe in the value and validity of the medicinal abilities of plants. This was, after all, given by the Creator himself and thus those who discredit its value should consider what our forebears since the very early days, used to treat fever, disease, and pain…. What after all is aspirin but the chemical equivalent of willow bark which was used in days long gone to treat pain and inflammation?

But back to running. Considering where I have been, this is indeed miraculous. Not a week goes by that I do not remember the statement by a neurologist that both my feet will eventually have to be amputated due to the irreversible nerve damage in my lower legs. Do I have news for that doctor!

Thankfully I never accepted, not for a second, that statement of doom. Now, when my legs are sore, I know it is from the exercise I did the day before. I have for quite a few years, been doing flexibility exercises (mostly Callanetics) to keep my muscles healthy. Then I expanded on this by running around a soccer pitch. Now I am running 5km every day. And doing so successfully. And am way past 100 Park Runs.

My training program is not extreme. It is, for all intents and purposes, a rather slow start. However, in line with my overall analytical approach, I am sure that taking it from this level is the intelligent way to go. What after all, would be the point of trying to prove something and injuring

TERMO DE RESPONSABILIDADE

Todas as estratégias e informações que você lerá neste livro e o que aprendi quando comecei a usar técnicas avançadas de acabamento para aumentar o valor de meus produtos são fruto de minhas experiências profissionais na área, além de mais de 15 anos de pesquisas científicas. pesquisa em fabricação aditiva (impressão 3D) e manufatura avançada.

Embora eu tenha feito o possível para garantir a precisão e a mais alta qualidade dessas informações, de modo que todas as técnicas e métodos ensinados aqui sejam altamente eficazes para qualquer pessoa que não esteja inclinada a aprender e faça o esforço necessário para aplicá-las conforme as instruções, esses métodos e informações não podem ser aprendidos teoricamente, mas apenas na prática.

As estratégias e informações apresentadas aqui são para todos, mas não para ninguém. Você precisa estar disposto. Além disso, sua situação específica pode não ser adequada perfeitamente aos métodos e técnicas ensinadas neste guia. Portanto, você pode usá-lo ajustando as informações de acordo com sua necessidade específica e, por esse motivo, os resultados podem variar de pessoa para pessoa. Não há garantia, há apenas uma experiência e testemunho de milhares de clientes bem-sucedidos graças a esse método.

INTRODUÇÃO

Acredito que este livro será muito útil para muitas pessoas. Por um lado, é extraordinário para quem já trabalha com serviços de impressão em 3D ou possui seus próprios negócios digitais em 3D. Por outro lado, este livro é ótimo para quem não trabalha com impressão 3D nem possui negócios digitais em 3D.

Além disso, as estratégias que expus aqui vão além e ajudam a criar uma infinidade de novos tipos de negócios. Portanto, tenho vários estudos de caso em diferentes segmentos, como assistência médica, aplicação médica, indústria, jogos, odontologia, design de produtos, manutenção, serviços, robótica, engenharia, arquitetura e muitos outros.

Ficarei muito feliz se você terminar este livro e perceber as múltiplas oportunidades e a potencial aplicação desta metodologia.

Na última parte deste livro, também apresentarei uma estratégia de produto que usei na minha empresa em ascensão. Essa estratégia é tão inacreditável que me permitiu:

- Tenha a maior margem de lucro que eu já vi no planeta
- Ter uma estrutura enxuta, com poucos funcionários (onde eu nem estava fisicamente presente a maior parte do tempo)

- Kickoff com um investimento tão pequeno que todos poderiam implementar
- Torne seus clientes extremamente felizes e fiéis
- Tenha excelentes resultados

Você descobrirá essa estratégia na terceira parte deste livro. Mas, primeiro, terei de lhe ensinar duas coisas muito importantes para entender por que essa estratégia é tão valiosa.

1. Qual é o tipo de qualidade (produto ou serviço) que seu cliente vê

Você aprenderá a usar, em seus negócios ou projetos pessoais, uma estratégia de fabricação que trará **resultados mensuráveis e quantitativos**.

Medir cada ação e projeto que você entregar permitirá que você **dimensione seu investimento** em um ambiente de risco super reduzido. Portanto, ajudará sua empresa a melhorar, além de criar novas filiais e novas oportunidades.

A melhor parte é que **você não precisa começar com um orçamento milionário**. Invista com sabedoria um orçamento muito pequeno é suficiente para melhorar seus projetos e aumentar os resultados.

Uma coisa que posso garantir é que, depois de terminar esta parte do livro, você nunca verá os serviços de impressão 3D do mesmo ponto de vista. Para 99% dos usuários de impressão 3D (iniciantes a especialistas), a fabricação avançada é uma grande caixa preta na qual você envia uma STL para um lado e recebe um objeto de impressão 3D do outro lado.

Depois de terminar esta parte do livro, você fará parte de 1% das pessoas que entendem o que acontece dentro da misteriosa caixa preta.

Depois de explicar isso para você, eu vou te ensinar:

2 NEM TODOS OS CLIENTES SÃO IGUAIS

Primeiro de tudo, você precisará entender que existem três tipos de clientes que você atenderá ou converterá. A compreensão desses clientes permitirá que você crie estratégias adequadas para satisfazer melhor suas necessidades ocultas essenciais. Portanto, é possível atingir o pico de eficiência para a maioria ou todos os clientes, de acordo com a flexibilidade da sua estratégia.

Tipos de Clientes

Vamos imaginar que todos os clientes são como um Iceberg. Na maioria das vezes, apenas a ponta do iceberg é visível (fora d'água). Nesse caso, a dica do iceberg ilustra nosso primeiro tipo de cliente. No entanto, esse cliente é o mais procurado entre os concorrentes, que pretendem convertê-lo e aumentar a fidelidade do cliente.

Bem, você deve ter imaginado que tipo de cliente é esse?

"As pessoas não sabem o que querem até que você as mostre. É por isso que nunca confio em pesquisa de mercado."

Steve Jobs

3 OS 2 MODELOS DE SERVIÇOS AVANÇADOS DE IMPRESSÃO 3D

Toda empresa, não importa em que estágio está (seja a que está dando passos de bebê ou a gigante do mercado), quer e precisa ter mais clientes.

Mas, para conseguir isso, o que geralmente é feito? As pessoas investem em equipamentos, marketing, mão de obra e infraestrutura. Em outras palavras, é senso comum que é necessário melhorar a qualidade e a produtividade para atrair mais clientes e criar um relacionamento de lealdade. E, claro, você quer isso, não é?

Serviços técnicos de Branding

Quando o assunto é fabricação avançada, o primeiro tipo de serviço de impressão 3D avançada que aparece em nossa mente geralmente se parece com isso:

Um enorme laboratório de fabricação, atendido por CNCs de alta velocidade de um lado, impressoras 3D cultivadas por FFF, DLP e SLA do outro lado, ao lado de uma gigante SLM (impressora 3D de objetos metálicos). Na parte traseira deste laboratório de fabricação avançado, um par de braços robóticos move objetos de um transportador para uma câmara de pintura automática. Nesse caso, tudo é controlado e gerenciado remotamente por uma inteligência artificial.

Você viu a imagem? Bem.

Nesta abordagem, o elemento técnico é predominante e, como conseqüência, espera-se que o objeto fabricado seja exatamente como especificado. Por acaso, o cliente ficará feliz no final da entrega do serviço. Essa abordagem é chamada de Serviços técnicos de Branding.

O principal problema dessa abordagem é que você precisa investir muito dinheiro para começar a ter bons resultados. E a pior parte é que você não pode nem medir os ganhos e as perdas desse investimento

Por que isso é um problema?

Como seu investimento se torna um valor de amortização nos custos fixos, enquanto seu cliente não espera pagar por esse investimento. Na opinião do cliente, sua qualidade não passa de uma obrigação.

Em contraste com empresas gigantes, as pequenas e médias empresas não têm milhões de dólares para investir em centros de fabricação avançados. Eles têm orçamentos apertados e cada centavo investido precisa ser compensado para não comprometer o negócio.

Obviamente, sabe-se que grandes empresas como GE, HP Solid Concept, Stratasys, sistemas 3D e MakerBot investem milhões de dólares em laboratórios de fabricação e serviços técnicos de marcas.

E essa abordagem funciona?

Sim. Caso contrário, eles não estariam fazendo.

A parte mais difícil é o fato de essas empresas subutilizarem esses equipamentos na verdade não sabem o ganho real obtido em seus laboratórios.

Você, como hobby ou proprietário de uma empresa de pequeno /

"Qualidade é mais importante que quantidade. Um home run é muito melhor do que dois duplos."

Steve Jobs

4 SERVIÇOS ORIENTADOS AO CLIENTE VS SERVIÇOS ORIENTADOS À QUALIDADE

Como você viu no capítulo anterior, os serviços direcionados ao cliente foram criados para medir, melhorar resultados e aumentar o impacto do recurso de valor nos clientes. Esses recursos podem aumentar o valor percebido de maneira incremental ou sensata. Em outras palavras, dependendo do tipo de recurso e estratégia que você usa, os resultados serão maiores.

No grupo de estratégias que implicam em valor percebido sensível, algumas etapas foram incluídas no processo para aumentar os resultados. Essa estratégia é chamada de serviços orientados à qualidade.

Deixe-me explicar melhor para você.

Na abordagem clássica, você produz objetos e entrega ao cliente de maneira direta. Portanto, o **valor percebido** é incluído no serviço em apenas uma etapa.

Por outro lado, os serviços orientados à qualidade afetam as 8 dimensões da **qualidade percebida** (elementos nos quais os clientes veem que vale a pena gastar seu dinheiro) em apenas **três etapas**.

com outro cliente que você tem controle.

Clientes Controlados

Desde as primeiras revoluções industriais, uma coisa é certa. O trabalho colaborativo e o design colaborativo garantiam que as manufaturas crescessem como satélite de seus clientes.

Por exemplo, as indústrias automotivas não são nada sem fábricas de motores ou de rodas.

Portanto, é possível dizer que um cliente controlado é aquele que **compartilha a responsabilidade do projeto e do design.**

Você entendeu o que eu vou chegar, não foi?

No momento em que você começa a ajudar seus clientes, você se torna o parceiro deles. Portanto, serviços orientados à qualidade começam a se tornar realidade.

Para atingir metas desafiadoras, são necessárias ferramentas poderosas. Vou apresentar a você as três ferramentas que permitirão que você entenda seu cliente controlado.

- 8 dimensões
- QFD - Casa de qualidade
- Experiência cega

8 Dimensões

De maneira geral, a qualidade percebida possui 8 dimensões,

- Dimensão 1: Desempenho
- Dimensão 2: Recursos
- Dimensão 3: Confiabilidade
- Dimensão 4: conformidade
- Dimensão 5: Durabilidade
- Dimensão 6: Facilidade de manutenção
- Dimensão 7: Estética

- Dimensão 8: Percepção

Como aprendemos, cada cliente vê o mundo de uma janela diferente, mas todos instintivamente prestam atenção a todas as dimensões, mesmo que essa dimensão não seja importante para eles.

O **desempenho** indica que o produto funciona da maneira que deveria funcionar. É importante observar que esse não é um assunto óbvio. Você deve considerar que, apesar dos erros no design do cliente, o sucesso do seu serviço dependerá de quão bem o produto funciona ou de quão bem as peças prototipadas são montadas.

Nesse caso, os testes experimentais fazem todo o sentido antes da entrega final.

Recursos são coisas que geram valor para o produto. Essa dimensão é a que você deve explorar mais.

Cada design possui características especiais para se tornar único. Cada designer também tem o seu.

Como os recursos são pequenas partes do design, você pode aprimorá-lo progressivamente e de forma incremental, como apresentamos na estratégia de serviços orientados ao cliente.

Confiabilidade são as coisas e os elementos que fazem seu cliente confiar e confiar em seus serviços. Essa é uma característica da marca definida fundamentalmente durante os primeiros serviços ou por indicação.

Nesse caso, os recursos que garantem a confiabilidade do seu produto fazem muita diferença.

Eu vou te dar um exemplo. Uma vez, implementei a política de entrega de um relatório de teste dimensional / de montagem / de tração no produto / peças de entrega. Nesse caso, o cliente

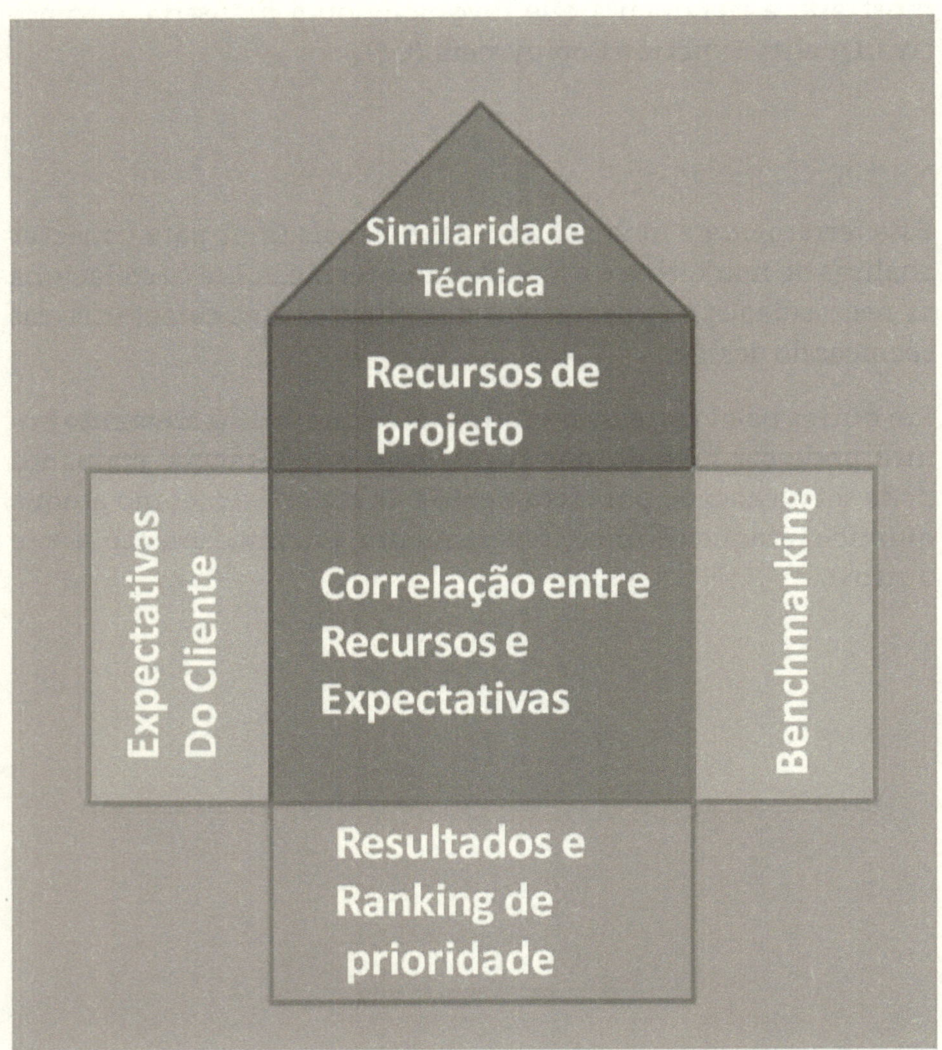

Similaridade Técnica
Recursos de projeto
Expectativas Do Cliente
Correlação entre Recursos e Expectativas
Benchmarking
Resultados e Ranking de prioridade

De uma maneira simples, o QFD pode ser descrito em 3 partes principais:

- Expectativas do cliente
- Características de design
- Correlação entre expectativas e recursos

Ilustrando a aplicação desta tabela, mostrarei a análise de uma Caneca simples que um cliente meu pediu minha ajuda para desenvolver.

Nesse caso, o cliente esperava que o Caneca fosse:

- grande
- Encaixe no suporte do carro
- Pareça com ele mesmo
- Não jogue café no carro por causa do movimento
- mão quente
- não queime as mãos
- Mantenha o café quente

Por outro lado, o que eu tinha na minha caixa de ferramentas para desenvolver este produto?

Eu poderia definir:

- Volume interno da caneca (Oz ou ml)
- Tamanho (pés cúbicos ou mm³)
- Cor
- Material
- Forma
- revestimento e pintura
- Isolamento
- tampa

Perfeito, sabendo a importância de cada expectativa do meu cli-

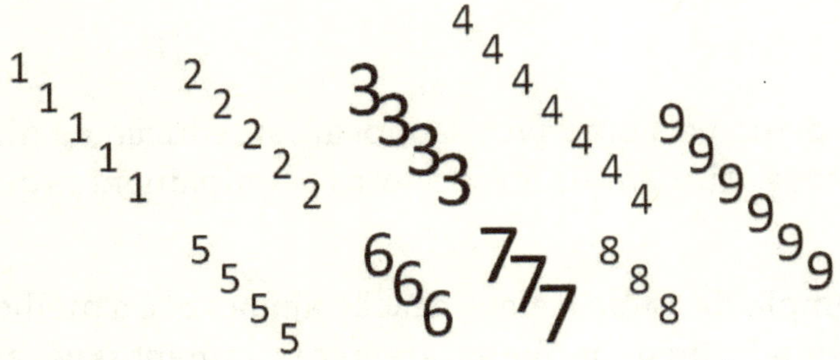

Para implementar esta etapa, ensinarei uma técnica rápida para que isso aconteça.

1)   Coloque tudo o que você usa em um só lugar (isso se tornará uma bagunça no começo, mas valerei a pena)

2)   Descarte todos os itens que você não usa há mais de 6 meses. Separe os itens que você não usa em dois meses e identifique-os com uma etiqueta vermelha. Coloque todos os itens marcados em vermelho em um canto.

3)   Classifique todos os itens úteis de acordo com a forma, aplicação e com que frequência você os utiliza. Identifique-os com etiquetas verdes, amarelas e cinza.

1)   Tags verdes são itens que você usa constantemente (mais de uma vez por dia)

2)   Tags amarelas são itens que você não usa com tanta

frequência (mais de uma vez por semana)

3)   Tags cinza são itens que você não usa com frequência (mais de uma vez por mês)

4)   Agora que você classificou os itens por frequência, forma e aplicação, coloque cada grupo em uma caixa

5)   Etiquetas verdes estarão próximas a você, enquanto etiquetas amarelas estarão na prateleira em uma posição acessível. As tags cinza estarão na prateleira em uma posição não acessível.

2º Passo (Organizar)

A ordem estabelecida está centrada no fato de que o fluxo de trabalho deve ser suave e rápido para reduzir a perda de tempo e aumentar a produtividade.

Os estágios básicos para alcançar uma boa organização são:

1)   Organize todos os itens necessários para facilitar a localização e o uso.

2)   Defina qual é o local mais curto para cada item ou grupo de itens que você usa no processo.

3)   Defina o local da correção para cada item e grupo. Cada item precisa ter seu próprio lugar.

Usando uma loja de impressão 3D simples como exemplo, mostrarei como o Set em ordem torna a fabricação mais ágil e rápida.

Imagine que você está produzindo objetos de impressão 3D em 3 estações de trabalho, onde uma delas é uma estação de pintura.

O fluxo de trabalho básico para cada parte geralmente segue:

1)   impressoras 3d
2)   Estação de acabamento
3)   estação de pintura
4)   câmara de secagem

Por exemplo, imagine a seguinte situação:

Você recebe um pedido de 70 produtos médios / semana em que cada parte consome:

- 10 horas em impressão 3D
- 2 horas em preparação e lixamento
- 2 horas em acabamento copo
- 10 min de primer de pulverização
- Primário de secagem de 30 min
- 10 min em pintura em primeira mão
- 20 min em secagem 1ª mão
- 10 min de pintura em segunda mão
- Pintura de secagem de 1 hora

Imagine que você tem 4 impressoras 3D trabalhando com capacidade total para você, além de contar com 3 pessoas em sua equipe.

Assim, o seu tempo takt será de 1,7 h / produto. Como conseqüência, você pode começar a analisar por sua configuração básica e depois equilibrar (compartilhar tarefas).

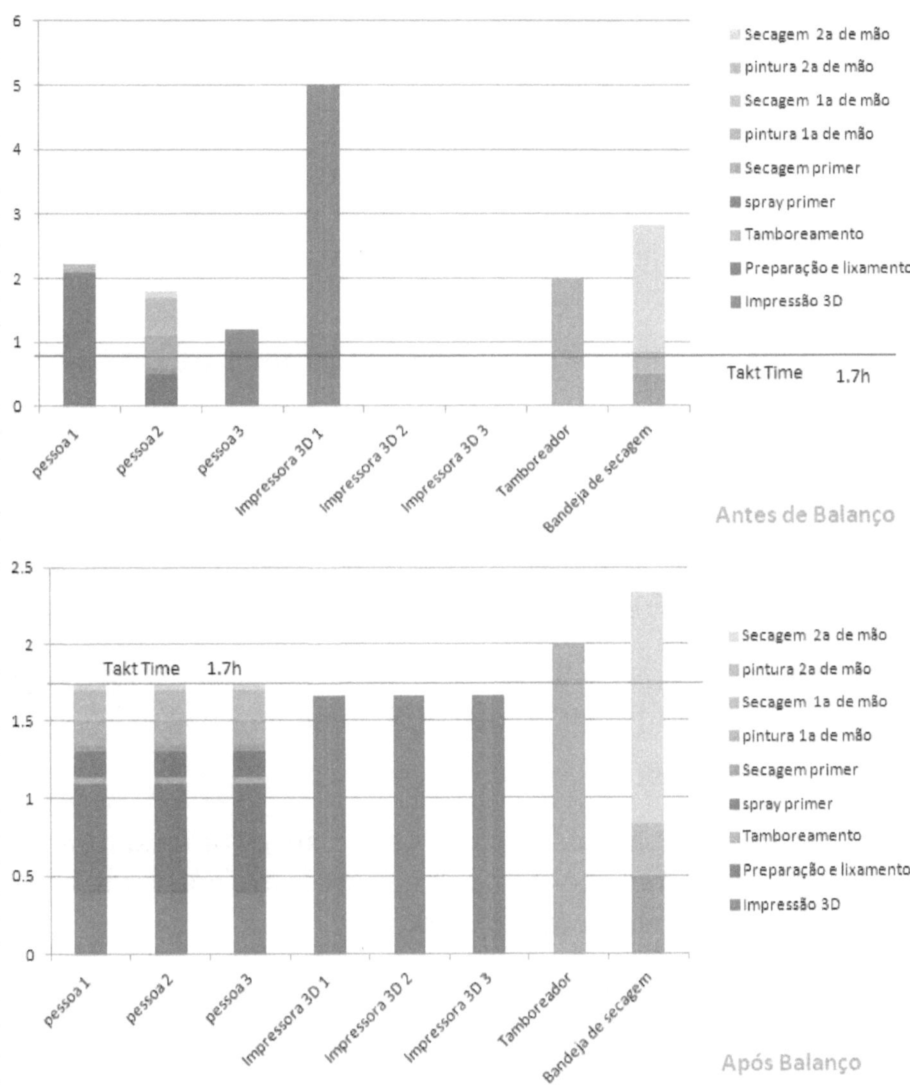

Neste exemplo, três impressoras 3D são suficientes para atender o tempo de Takt e, após o equilíbrio, as mesmas três pessoas também são suficientes.

Técnicas avançadas de acabamento (o Santo Graal)

A terceira técnica é o que chamei de "Santo Graal" da fabricação de impressão 3D. Esta é uma estratégia que é de longe a que mais traz resultados para mim e meus clientes.

PARTE 3

DESEJA VOAR MAIS
ALTO ? APRENDA A
CRIAR UM LABORATÓRIO
DE ALTA TECNOLOGIA
E BAIXO CUSTO

◆ ◆ ◆

"Qualidade é dar aos clientes o que eles querem."

Sam Walton

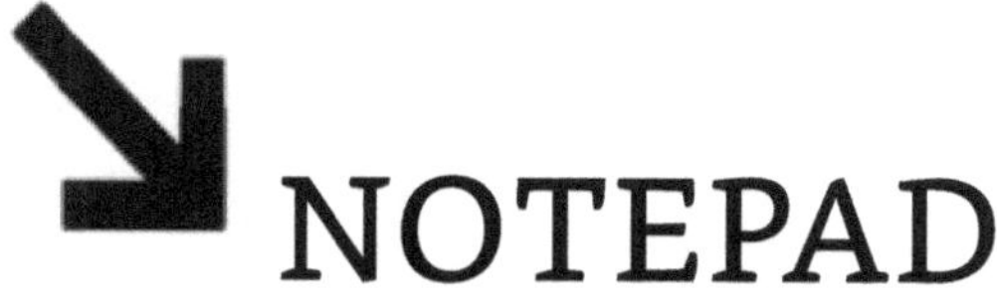

NOTEPAD

birthday cake!" Right then and there... I knew you was the coolest female ever. Because if you was mad that I bought back the wrong kind of ice cream, you didn't let your anger show! But I have a secret to tell you! I picked the Sorbet ice cream out of all the other flavors, because I never had that kind of ice cream before... and wanted it bad, because the colorful design on the box made it look like it was good. But I've learned that it didn't go well with birthday cake at all. So there you have it! Todda... You were always smart! Like your intelligence was at a level out of this world! You bought me my first video game system... the first Nintendo. And my first Hawaiian short set! My first Big Mac sandwich from McDonalds. It's crazy that I can remember the most littlest things that meant so much to me growing up! Most of all I want to thank you, for being one of my great big sisters! I love you always, no matter what! Schrise... it's been wonderful, all the years we've grown to do the things that most people wouldn't dare! We have so many memories, good... bad... ugly, whatever they wanna label it. But I know one thing! "Kit-Kat" is ALWAYS gonna be my sister no matter what. F#*$ the haters. Keep your head up high Ma! You know the count... I love you big sis! Anne... Thanks! For holding it down and believing in me.I told you that I was gonna put my talent to use. This is only the beginning... watch me work! I love you sis! Jennifer... spit a few bars for me, so I can turn up! You could of been the female rapper, that took the game to a whole different level. You know that music sh%$ runs in the family! But times change... and so does people, places, and things! But it's been a minute since we connected, so just know that I'm bout to be greater than I ever was. And hopefully everyone can land in a comfortable position. I love you lil sis! Sharon... I'm starting to believe that your half Mexican and Jamaican! LOL. You work all the time... I can't even remember the last time that I've seen you, or heard from you! Just know that I'm elevating! I love you lil sis! Alexandria Miller... it's been too long since we last seen or heard from one another! But I promise you that we will find each other again! I love you lil sis! To my 2 brothers Bo and Curtis Mitchell. Bo... I'm not gonna even get into all the talking, I often tend to say less... 'cause I've seen and done a lot! Just know that you my n%##@ 4life! You introduced me to my first pair of Nikes, and my first gold chain... and they wonder how my swagg got retarded! I got it from my brother! "Facts!" This is for you bro... I finally did something positive! Love u 2 death my G! NEVER 4 GET IT!!! "I am my brother's keeper!" Curtis...it's been year's man... too many year's, but I'll find you eventually! I love you bro... and can't wait to see you just to catch up on things! Most importantly, always know that I will never forget about you! To: My Ace... "Giavonni", Bayonne,Nj. (For always being authentic, it gets no realer than that! Bet you thought I forgot about you! Love you always Ma!) To: "Anissa", Bayonne, Nj. For the moments shared, that hold special memories! To: "Victoria", Norfolk, Va. For being the true definition of a friend and making time to listen... when nobody else would. You are appreciated! To: D. "Harlem Boi Nique" Thompson. Portsmouth, Va. I would never forget about you my n%##@... stay motivated, stay focused, and always stay true! When I rise... we rise together! No new friends... and F*#$ them b%#@*-$, hold ya head up! Most of them lie, because they did things in life... that they don't want revealed."FACTZ!" 1Luv my n%##@. To: My brutha from another! D. "Head" Hammon. Norfolk, Va. Our journey was one, that was built out of loyalty and respect! And commitment to doing greater in life! Owning anything in this world... means nothing without hard work and dedication. You learn to appreciate and value it's worth more... when you get it out the mud! 1Luv my n%##@.) To: Ms. Pamela Noble. Richmond, Va. I gave you my word that I wouldn't forget about you, and shout you out! And I'm giving you the opportunity to read my work! Hopefully you enjoyed it, being that you love reading! And will enjoy all the many projects that's next to come! Thank You for the support!) To: Ms. Lynn Noble. Richmond, Va. You're one of the most sweetest people that I've ever met! You're very down to earth, and cool like a fan! Thank You! For not judging me!) To: Ms. Ariel Noble. Richmond, Va. (For all the laughs, and great conversations... the motivation, inspiration, and dedication of you, being that filter I needed to shake ALL the bulls%#@ off my shoulders! For being the "Beautiful Queen", that you truly are... and for being the biggest s%#$ starter that I know! (LOL) Laugh Out Loud. It's all about showing and proving, and you've earn your crown! "The Queen!" Love you genuinely... cause I would only be lying, if it was anything less! Most of all... Thank You for keeping it 1000 plus some, since day one! You're very special and beautiful! Don't never let no one tell you anything different! Stay elevated Ma! To: My young n%##@ D'Sean aka Lil D. Lancaster,Va. I've shown you... what it's like, to be in a pool full of sharks, and still be victorious! Sound bites mean nothing! It's a bigger picture when you focus and find your way. If you don't go within, you go without! "FACTZ!" You know what time it is... Loyalty is key! Shout out to my hood..."DUNCAN PROJECTS". "THE OLD DUNCAN"...and "THE NEW DUNCAN". The concrete jungle is historic... To all my N%##@'z, and my all my Women, it's too many of y'all to name everyone! Just know that I represented for the jects! To my original "G.L.P" (Get Large Posse) N%##@'z..... To All my fallen soldiers, " Gone But Never 4 Gotten!" Shout out... To the whole Jersey City! Every project's, street, corner, block, and Ave. "Marion Projects!" "G.S.T" "Gun Shot Towers!" aka (Montgomery Projects). "The old Curry woods Projects!"... and the "New!" "Lafayette Projects!" "Booker T. Projects!" "The New Houses!" "16th.St. Projects!" Shout out... To the whole "Bayonne!" aka "Budahville!" Shout out...to the whole "Brick City!" (Newark). "Irvington!" "East Orange!" "Hoboken!" NEW JERSEY PERIOD!!! STAND UP!! BROOKLYN,NY. STAND UP!! DELAWARE... STAND UP!! VIRGINIA... STAND UP!! To: My nephews... Dannan aka Flip Deniro, Malcom, (R.I.P Kareem), Jonathan, and Mario. And To My nieces: Leslie, Indigo, Xiomara, Natasha, Halajiah, and Karizma. I remember the moments when you all were babies... and learning how to crawl and walk! Now almost all of you are grown, and living your lives! Time fly's within the blink of any eye! I love you all and miss everyone very much! To: My BROOKLYN n%##@'z..... "Bless", "Mizz", " Wise", & "Wiz". To My Rasta n%##@... BLESS aka Rude Boy. Staying humble is something I've learned, by doing the knowledge to you! In order to understand the people, you have to first be able to identify, then speak their language! It's amazing how one mans pain, can become another man's strength! Yea...Yea! To: Mizz, You gave me one of the truest builds ever! "N%##@'z are like a deck of cards... you have to watch n%##@'z, cause eventually they'll expose their hand". And that conversation was at the poker table. 1Luv my n%##@. To: A. Brembray aka The God Wise... We connected on

Sitting in his truck scrolling through his phone, Nice was punch drunk by the screen shots Treasure sent him. He had literally been staring at her fuckin pussy all day! Treasure was in fact, just that, A Treasure! A half Jamaican and Indian amazon out of Bridgeport, CT who took a liking to Nice. Not because he tipped well cuz all the strippers knew the tippers, but because he conducted himself like a professional, and not like most thirsty ass niggaz do when they throw a couple of ones. Treasure's hopes were high that maybe Nice will one day make her his. Her mind was set on nothing other than swallowing his dick, then winding on it like she was at a reggae fest. Reading the text that just scrolled across the top of his screen, "bout to slide through". Nice replied "copy", then looked at another pussy shot of Treasure squirting like a water fountain. "Dammnnn!!!" He said out loud to himself before tucking the phone in his pocket. A few minutes had passed before Don Smoke pulled up beside the all black on black Range Rover Sport, sitting on 30's.

Nice rolled down his passenger's side window, then leaned over to holla at Don. "What's happening my nigg? You already know the count big bro." Don answered. "Look. I need you to cook this chicken and get it to Gi-Gi for me A.S.A.P. I been on the road plus moving around in the city. Ain't had time to do shit for real. Plus i'm hungry as fuck and tired." "Say less bro." Nice replied!

Waking up to nothing but the blue pair of Cavalli jeans laying on the edge of the bed. Bliss couldn't help but to wonder, where the fuck her man was at now! Quickly getting up on her feet out the bed, she stood in pure perfection. Her honey comb shaped breast were full with nipples that resemble milk duds, and her thighs were as firm as sweet potatoes. Without a doubt. Bliss had a bomb ass body, with long wavy jet black hair and all the features to accommodate her beauty. Noticing the sounds of running water, she headed to the bathroom where she saw Kiem standing under the shower head with his eyes closed. Paying no attention to his fist balled up, instead focusing on his dick that hung like no other. Her juices started to flow, as she began to massage herself. Rubbing her clitoris gently while sliding one finger, then two fingers deep inside her made her turn straight animal. She quickly pushed her left titty up to her mouth and popped her nipple inside and began sucking on it like crazy while shifting her two fingers around vigorously. inside her steaming wet pussy! Turned on by the presence of a real nigga, a real big dick nigga. Bliss quietly crept into the shower with Kiem and got down on her knees. She slowly took every inch of him deep into her moist hot mouth, until she had nothing but balls on her lips. Kiem opened his eyes and let out a sigh of relief, as Bliss worked her throat like she was singing for an opera. Still popping her own pussy, she handled her mans' dick like a full-time job, because it was her job to take care of him completely.

With her legs trembling at the peak of her climax, she came long and hard all over her fingers. Bliss had her way with Kiem, and with one slow deep suck she had the head of his dick on her tonsils. As he released every bit of himself deep down her throat.

Kiem got weak legged and had to hold himself up on the shower walls. Once he regained his strength, he pulled Bliss up to him and held her in his arms tightly.

After bathing, they both exited the shower, handled the rest of their personal hygiene then

proceeded to get dress. Kiem sent Don Smoke a text "meet me at the canton in 30mins., R.N.S." (Real Nigga Shit). While entering the lock code,
Don Smoke got a text from Kiem. After
reading it, he instantly hit back "O.M.W." Once the floor compartment ejected, Don grabbed the kilo and handed it through his driver's side. I'm on it now bro. Nice replied. I'll hit you up later, we probably bounce to Club Angel's tonight. Got this bad amazon on deck, plus she got some freaks that do what it do!" "Aight, make sure you get at me. We lit! Don Smoke stated. They saluted each other before pulling off turning in different directions.
After tying up the leather white and infra-red retro #6 Jordan's, Kiem then put on his matching track jacket before calling out to Bliss. "Ma! Come on, we gotta make moves. Ya ass stay flyer than me, and you still take hours getting dressed". "Boyyeee!! Shut ya mouth." Bliss replied, before appearing in an all red one piece pants suit, which hugged every curve on her body. Fascinated by her beauty, Kiem did the honors with helping Bliss buckle the straps on her red leather open toe Gucci sandals. Bliss was a hundred so labels didn't matter. She could put on some shit straight out of K-mart and set a fashion trend. It's no wonder why most niggaz envied Kiem. It wasn't just because of his money; it was because he had money and a bad bitch too! "Thank You!" Bliss replied. As Kiem pulled her close to him and said. "you're special, anything for you ma". Then gently kissed her the on lips. "So what you think?" Bliss asked referring to her outfit. "Amazing. simply amazing!" Kiem stated. Then grabbed her by both of her two French braided ponytails, which hung down deep her back passing her ass cheeks. "Come on beautiful, walk so I can see that ass bounce " Bliss loved the way Kiem handled her, especially whenever he grabbed her by her hair. That was his signature touch! Tucking the .45 in his waistline, Kiem then grabbed his white and red bulls snapback off the wall hat rack. All while still holding Bliss by her ponytails. They exited the condo and made way down the hallway to the elevator, without looking back at the pried open lock on the door. Now on the elevator Kiem asked "you hungry?" "Yeessss. I'm starved." Bliss replied.

Reaching the first floor, Kiem took Bliss by the hand and escorted her out of the elevator, and into the lobby, then out the front entrance of the condominiums. Approaching both their cars that was parked next to each other. Kiem stated. we taking the 550SL! You driving Bliss asked? Nah sexy. you got the wheel. Kiem answered. Go to the Canton ma!

Meanwhile riding down Kennedy Blvd, Nice was on his way to holla at Gi-Gi, so he can cook the chicken for her. Gi-Gi was part of their squad. She handled all the work that was flat footed with only a selected few individual that trapped for her within her city. Gi-Gi was from Bayonne, NJ aka Boodaville and was well known, especially once she started getting money. Her and Kiem had met back in the day when Kiem was wanted in Jersey City and had to switch locations, because police was down on his top. Gi-Gi was his ace and although they never fucked around with each other they were both shy to admit how much they really liked one another. As time grew and their

Kiem of the lock situation on his door. "Mr. Pairings, I received a call today about a possible breaking and entering from one of your neighbors as they returned home and noticed the lock on your door open. I haven't notified authorities as of yet, because I was on my way to the office to pull your phone number off file. But I will quickly notify authorities so that you can file a report and notify them of any belongings that might have been taken from your residence. Kiem instantly interjected the idea of Ms. Estelvo calling the police and stated." Ms. Estelvo, I apologize, I truly do! But there's no need for authorities. You see when I got home from the bar, it was only then that I realized I had lost my keys and couldn't gain access to my condo. With no other way inside, I went out to my car and got a screwdriver and pried the lock open. Ms. Estelvo grinned deviously cuz she knew he was blowing smoke up her ass, but she loved it cuz she now had him where she wanted him at. "However, I will pay the repair fee to have the lock replaced, well as labor!" Kiem stated. "No need Mr. Pairings." Ms. Estelvo replied. While she grinned seductively looking at Kiem. "I'll call and have a new lock installed and as little as an hour." Ms. Estelvo said. "Thank You!" Kiem stated. No problem she replied as she opened her legs only to reveal the phatest camel toe that Kiem has ever seen sitting underneath her purple lace panties as she stood up from her chair. Don Smoke couldn't believe the bullshit talk, plus what he just seen with his own eyes. As him and Kiem walked out of the office, his blood started to boil as they made way towards the elevator. Stepping inside. Don shout out aggressively." Bro that bitch ain't right I was watching her the whole damn time, she knows something 'bout your spot being hit. Just think the owner of an expensive condominium property, received a call from one of your neighbors about a possible breaking and entering and ain't nobody call the cops yet! Bullshit!!!" Don Smoke said out loud. "This is a high-priced residential area, twelve would of flooded this whole neighborhood looking for a suspect. Then the bitch spread her legs wide open for you, as she got up from her chair. My nigga! She had straight lust in her eyes for you, the whole time she been talking!" Don Smoke stated. "She ain't never try to give you the pussy?" Don 'Smoke asked. Kiem looked at Don thinking hard about the question, then said. "Yo the lady has been down on a nigga ever since I bought the condo". In fact, I remember when me and Bliss came to view the place and I introduced Bliss as my woman. Ms. Estelvo was on some real drama shit!" Kiem stated. She was acting like she was my bitch and Bliss posed a threat to her wellbeing. She even gave me a box of Hidden Treasure, Grand Toro Cigars as a gift once I purchased the place. I don't even fuck with cigars, but she insisted that I accept the gift as and taken of our business and future friendship. I didn't think nothing of it, until we were leaving and Bliss walked out first. As I followed behind something was like turn around. So I suddenly turned back and seen shorty flash me her titties. I ain't gone even lie, them titties was sitting up nice. I knew the bitch was on some real freak shit. But if Bliss caught her ass flashing me anything, that would have been straight havoc! I had a few run ins with her here and there, but nothing spectacular to as though we fucked. The broad basically harassed me out to dinner, paid the bill, bought me a gem set Rolex because she said that I looked like a man that demanded respect. So it's a must that I acquire exquisite taste to accommodate my style, and she had the perfect gift for me. At first, when I saw the box I was like kool another roley. But when I opened it. I was like damn!!! A rainbow-bezel rose-gold Daytona. And I ain't even fuck this bitch. And then one day, she even pulled up on me mysteriously out of nowhere while I was serving Nicco three birds. She ain't see me handled business, or nothing like that 'cuz the exchange between us was done, by time she rolled up. But other than her having a like for the kid, I don't think she know anything about my crib getting hit or the money and drugs that was in it" "Yo! 750k plus 100 brickz. Somebody is all the way up right now!" Don Smoke stated. As Kiem gritted his teeth in anger cuz he knew Don's statement was the truth. "And where's the watch she bought you?" Don Smoke asked Kiem. "It's in my main safe with my other my other drip, and money that I now have to pay the connect with. Stepping off the elevator they both paced down the hallway to the front door of the condo, as Kiem pointed to the lock on the door and jokingly said. " This is what my drunk ass did". They both laughed and walked through the door. Heading straight to the bedroom walk in closet. Kiem removed a section of the carpet, which revealed the floor safe that had been drilled open. Without hesitation Don Smoke said to Kiem, "Bro this had to be an inside job. Look at how perfect the drill hole is, plus the fine pieces of shard metal scattered around from the drilling. Not to mention the fact, no one would have ever thought about a floor safe being exactly where you had it at. But who the fuck could have known about the floor safe, besides the company that installed it, for it to be an inside job?" Kiem asked. Now that's what we have to find out! Don Smoke answered. Grabbing the cream-colored Gucci duffle bag off the closet floor, Kiem snatched the pair of cream-colored Alejandro Ingelmo sneakers off his shoe rack and put 'em inside the duffel. Then grabbed his burgundy Dior jacket and pants, and cream color Lavin t-shirt and stuffed the clothes inside before he zipped the duffel bag close. With nothing valuable left in the condo besides some electronics, furniture, and designer, Kiem and Don Smoke exited the place. Taking the main stairway this time all the way down to the lobby floor. They both made way through the stairway entrance heading down the lobby hallway. when Ms. Estelvo had stopped them right in front of the lobby desk. "Mr.Pairings" she called out. "I just wanted to inform you that Ario will be back to work momentarily, and he will have the new set of keys for you, once the new lock has been installed." "Thank You!" Kiem stated as him and Don continued past the lobby desk and out into the parking lot. Kiem touched the sensor under his break light on the trunk, and the trunk opened instantly as he tossed the duffle bag inside. Looking at Don he then said "You know what time it is. We own Thursday nights! But tonight is gone be epic. You know we usually throw 30k on stage for the ladies, but we upping the ante tonight. We throwing 100k up in that bitch!" "Say no more." Don replied, before telling Kiem. "You crazy as fuck! But I see ya vision. Big bank takes little bank." Kiem smiled 'cuz he knew Don Smoke understood his machination. "Yo! I gotta make way to this connect, plus check on Bliss. After I handle things and get situated, Imma hit ya phone so we can link up and bounce!" Kiem stated. They saluted each other which was a code of loyalty amongst their cipher, before getting into their cars and parting ways. With seventy-two ounces of straight drop (crack) individually bagged up and ready to go. Gi-Gi separated thirty of the ounces into sets of five, before placing them into six different heavy-duty zip lock bags. She then divided of the crack down to the size of mini chips. Watching her girls go to work, Gi-Gi made it known that they we're all gone drip at "Main Event".

"Oh yea! This nigga Nicco is throwing a party at Main Event next Friday, and he got the nerve to be talking shit like he super authentic! I know y'all ain't hear nothing 'bout it, 'cuz I just caught wave. But "The 7 Sexes" will be Main Event biggest feature of the night!". "How the hell this nigga throwing a party at the city's best?" Rose XL asked. Before Gi-Gi could even respond to the question. Passion and N.D.A. both said at the same damn time, "who gives a fuck! "That nigga gettin' a lil change, now he wanna ball out of control. Shiittt.let him!" Passion Shooter stated. "He still wack as fuck, with his grimy disrespectful ass. I don't like the bitch!" Rose XL angrily stated as they all took shots at the nigga! "Look.I gotta fly! Y'all know what it is." Gi-Gi stated. Main Event drip hard!!

Parked down at the pier, patiently waiting in the back seat of the stretch limo, Karma decided to please herself until her appointment arrived. Opening her Mac book, she quickly went to her photos which revealed digital rotating pictures of Kiem. Having no panties on, she spread her legs wide open to reveal her neatly shaved pussy. With her juices flowing, she sucked hard on her middle finger, building up anticipation while staring at Kiem's pictures. Hot and bothered by her own train of thought, she slid her middle finger down to her pussy and started rubbing her clit like it was no tomorrow. Biting on her bottom lip while she played inside her, made her hotter than fish grease. Oh God! God. Fuck! She yelled out in pure ecstasy, as her legs trembled, and she climaxed all over her fingers. Breathing heavily from such a rush, she blew a kiss at Kiem's photo, then said "before it's all over with, you will be mine." Pulling the box of wet wipes from the console, she cleaned herself up then looked at her Cartier only to notice that her appointment was late. Keeping her composure, she sucked her teeth as she seen Forest Green 370z pull up. Closing the Mac book, her appointment approached the Continental then got inside. The conversation began with a scolding. "Nicco, you're late darling! Business is not conducted on these kinds of terms. A businessman conducts himself accordingly with all scheduled time appointments. Maybe you need to seek services elsewhere, being that you cannot follow instructions!" Karma boldly stated. "When I deal, I deal business that's beyond professional,100% A grade." "My fault Karma! I ran late behind getting the oil changed in my car." Nicco replied. "Getting the oil changed in your car". Karma repeated sarcastically! Ha! She laughed then continued talking. "Darling that is not a car! What you have is a ride, you need to advance your game. A car is luxury! That piece of shit is just a ride." Salty that a bitch just told him to his face, that his car ain't shit, he wanted to slap fire from her ass. Instead, he sucked it up and mixed it with a lot of ass kissing, to try and advance. "Karma, you did me a favor back when police pulled me, and I was riding dirty. It was either wear a fed case, or tell 'em where I got the drugs from, and I wasn't going to jail for possession of 3 kilos of cocaine. So.I cooperated with authorities, so I can walk free. I mean. at the end of the day, fuck Kiem!" Nicco said hatefully. "If the Feds watching him, fuck him! That nigga got enough paper to serve a life sentence." Nicco laughed! Karma smiled to herself devilishly at Nicco's statement about Kiem having enough paper to serve a life sentence. Cuz little did he know. Kiem was now broke! "That safe you just emptied out belonged to the man whom I desire and want more than the air that I breathe". Karma said to herself. Which was all to her advantage. Her plan was working precisely how she intended it to." Break the nigga pockets, and he will come to me. He will come and work for me then he will become my personal pleasure". "But on a more serious note, I do appreciate the help of your lawyer friend getting the charges dropped for illegal search procedure, before the charges even got processed. Besides, I'd be dead right now if the streetz found out I was a rat!! I wouldn't be getting no kind of money, no pussy, no nothing! But all that's 'bout to change thanks to you!" Nicco desperately said. "Two hundred and fifty thousand in cash and 100 brickz!! You put me on to the lick of a lifetime, and all I have to do is flood the city at the cheapest rate. "No darling." Karma interrupted. "This is where you lack ability to comprehend business. I gave you a get out jail free card. I gave you information and access to more money than you ever had in your life. I gave you power of position in these streetz with more drugs than you ever seen. I own you." Karma harshly stated. "Bitch! What the fuck you mean you own me?" Nicco snapped back asking. "I did you a favor, so the score is even. All that you own me shit?! Nah!" "Listen, you bastard! Your choice of words could very well be the end of your demise. So I suggest you watch your mouth darling before I have your tongue cut the fuck out! Do you understand, darling?" Karma sarcastically asked. Nicco nodded his head but deep down he wanted to knock this bitch head off for talking to him like he was a nobody! Although the streetz didn't fuck with him 'cuz he was a grimy ass nigga, things were gonna change once he started moving the cocaine. But he knew that he had another task at hand, which any nigga would consider a fair exchange for the 250k and 100 brickz, but what he didn't know is that he sold his soul to the devil. Reaching into her purse, she pulled out an envelope and gave it to him. As he opened the envelope and removed it's contents, it revealed a photo of Bliss. Stunned by the photo, it was only then that he realized that it was Kiem's girl, who he unknowingly agreed to murder. Deep in thought, Nicco knew all that good pussy was about to go to waste. "Everybody knew Bliss was a bad bitch! 5'2 with nice size titties, a small waist, and a phat ass. Her physique had to be about 32-28-40. Not to mention her long wavy jet black hair, and almond shaped eyes. "Shiittt.I wouldn't min d fucking the bitch before she die." Nicco said lustfully to himself. Looking into Karma eyes he knew that he couldn't back out of this one. Tearing the picture in half, he tossed the remains next him onto the seat and said "Consider it done." "Lovely darling!" Karma excitedly stated. Clinching her teeth she stared coldly into Nicco's eyes. "Contact me once this situation is executed." Karma seriously demanded. "I got you." Nicco replied while the snake in him said different. "Good darling. Now you're comprehending business. See your way to the trunk and you will find your power of position." Karma stated. Exiting the back of the stretch Continental, Nicco made his way towards the trunk as it opened revealing the army duffle bag. Snatching the duffle with both hands, he quickly moved towards the 370z and threw the bag into the back seat before getting into the car and pulling off. Speeding away, Nicco thought to himself that everything was 'bout to be heaven for him.100 brickz and in her pussy while still laying on her back, the second stripper measured the candy cane with the ruler, as she counted out loud. "Ten inches", "eleven inches", "one foot", "two feet". "Two fucking feet!!!" The stripper yelled out to the crowd. Mutha fuckas went crazy including the bitches! This is what everybody was waiting to see. Money was thrown all across the stage, while the second stripper inserted the candy cane up inside Treasure's pussy. Twisting her hips while grinding her ass on the floor, Treasure counted down out loud, while moaning. "Five, four, three, two, one". As the candy cane popped out of her soaking wet pussy. Only this time she was squirting like a water fountain. Her juices shot up in the air and left the crowd in awe!! Nice stood to his feet and made it "thunderstorm" on stage. "Thank You Daddy! Thank You!" Treasure excitedly stated. Pointing to his watch, she knew that he had to make way, as she whispered, "call me". Nodding his head in agreement, Nice, Kiem, Don Smoke, and Gi-Gi made way for the exit. Everyone dapped Big Dream up, as they walked out through the club's lobby and ready to exit the door. "Catch y'all next Friday, y'all be safe out there!" Big Dream said to the squad. Holding Gi-Gi by her waist, Kiem gave her a quick rundown, as he escorted her to her truck. "Look Ma! This what it is. That cash you got hold of? Split it amongst you and the rest of the Sexes." "Are you serious?" Gi-Gi asked. "Yea Ma!" Kiem replied. "We 'bout to make moves in a couple different states. You and the sexes are still going to be operating from y'all destinations. Only thing is there is going to be more product, which means more money for everybody!" Gi-Gi hugged Kiem so tight, that her skirt lifted revealing the lower part of her buttocks. Palming both of her ass cheeks as he hugged her back, they looked onto each other's eyes with infinite possibilities of what might could happen between them in bed. "Oh yea! I forgot to mention that Nicco offered Pink Bands ten thousand to fuck. When she wasn't with it, he still tossed the cash at her and told her to clean herself up. That's when she found out that he was having the party at Main Event and told her to be there and to bring her boss, and all that other bullshit 'bout moving for the low." Gi-Gi stated. Kiem then kissed Gi-Gi on her forehead, then said "fuck that nigga ma! We not worrying 'bout dude, what he doing, or what he got. But check! It don't hurt to conversate with the nigga and see what's good. Now get ya ass up in this truck, go home and get some rest! Here 'fore I forget". Pulling her black silk panties out of his pocket, she blushed as he placed 'em in her hand. "Love you nigga!" Gi-Gi stated. "Love you back Ma!" Kiem replied. She then started the Aviator and slowly pulled off. Back with Don Smoke and Nice, Nice said to Kiem, "you might as well fuck her, she ain't gone stop being flirtatious 'til you dick her down". "Nah bro! It's bigger than the pussy. You must be the sole controller of all things. If I know she's chasing the dick and I give it to her, that means I'm revolving around her universe. The sun don't rotate around the earth my nigga!" Kiem expressed. "Besides she just be playing, we comfortable with each other like that." Kiem stated. "Playing lil bro?". Nice replied. As him and Don Smoke laughed at Kiem's statement. "Whatever nigga y'all know the count" Kiem said arrogantly. "Yo, I'm 'bout to skate, gotta make a few stops before I hit Treasure up. Shit was crazy tonight. the bitches got to that bag on site!" Nice stated. "They always do." Don Smoke replied. "But my main man stole the show with his own private dancer." Don Smoke said. Everyone laughed as Nice saluted Kiem and Don

Smoke before getting into the Range. Watching the Black Monster fade into the shadow of the night, Don Smoke noticed that a crowd of niggaz been watching 'em since they exited the club. "We got attention my boyee!" He said to Kiem, while twisting a backwood. "Already." Kiem replied. As he took notice to the same crowd of niggaz that been eyeing 'em, sitting on the hood of Don's Audi, they blew the blunt of kush and focused on their surroundings. Two Dred Head niggaz and a short fat bald head nigga, approached Don Smoke and Kiem. "Yah Mon! Ye hav any herbs me buy?" One of the dread head niggaz asked. "Nah my dude! This right here is personal." Kiem replied. "Ye wan good smoke. Mee hav thee best Ganja 'round." The short fat bald head nigga said. 'Show 'em Store." One of the dreads reached in his jacket, then quickly froze like an ice sickle as Kiem and Don Smoke both drew their hammers down on the three men. "Don't move my nigga, and you won't have to become a T-shirt!" Kiem seriously stated. "Rass clot time ye deal rude boy! Mee nah wan no problems u shottos." Crrack!!! That was the next sound heard as Don Smoke's gun crashed against the fat Jamaican's temple, knocking him out cold. Blood gushed from the fat man's head, as his body laid motionless on the concrete. Checking the fat nigga for any weapons, Don Smoke took a Taurus G25 from his back pocket then rolled him over on his face. After making sure he was clean, Don Smoke quickly searched the first dread head nigga, then made him lay face down on the concrete with his hands on his head. The second dread head nigga started speaking in tongues, that it pissed Kiem off 'cuz he knew these mutha fuckas we're trying to line 'em up. "Move and ya a dead man!" Kiem stated while him and Don Smoke both had the dread at gun point. Unzipping his jacket, a Mac11 hung from a shoulder strap, which made it easy to carry and conceal. "Ahh my nigga! This the best Ganja round huh!" Kiem said sarcastically before snatching the Mac free from its shoulder strap. "Yo let's blow this spot 'fore twelve pull up". Kiem said. "Say less." Don replied. Getting into the R8 he heard four shots ring out. "Pop, pop, pop, pop!" Don knew it was Kiem who let 'em off. Seeing the dread head nigga fall to the ground screaming, blood squirted out both of his knees. While Kiem hopped in the Benz and pulled off, like if nothing never happened. Throwing the Audi in gear, Don Smoke was right behind him. as they caught every light going back downtown towards the Holland Tunnel.

    Back in Jersey City and still behind Kiem, Don Smoke hit his high beams three times. This was a signal they used to meet up at Don Smoke's spot. Going in their own direction, they split up temporarily only to meet again within 10mins. Pulling up on Vroom St, Don waited for Kiem to pull up before getting out the car. Looking through his rearview. he seen the purple machine bend the corner, as he hopped out the Audi and waited for Kiem to park. Tucking the Mac inside his jacket underneath his left arm, Kiem got out the car and walked towards Don as they both entered the building and went upstairs. When they entered the living room, they examined both guns that came with the game, free of charge. "Yea man we two guns up now!" Don Smoke said in a fake Jamaican accent as him and Kiem laughed. "My nigga! I don't know who the fuck them islanders thought we were." Kiem said harshly. "Money and bloodshed are the two things that people respect in this world. You can't just have a one track mind and expect shit to go smooth. There has to be some type of balance." Kiem explained retrieving a bottle of stated. "Girl what I'm a do with you?! "Anything you want. Just don't hurt me!" Bliss replied. "Copy!!" Kiem replied back then headed to the shower.

Sitting at the kitchen table drinking a can of 211Steel Reserve, Joany hit her last push, but still believed that it was another as she poked at her stem with a wire clothes hanger. Aggressively shoving the chore boy (copper wool) from one end to the other, she took her lighter and set fire to the stem as it burned nothing but the chore boy. Exhaling the black smoke, she grew irritated and searched the kitchen table, then the floor looking for a bump (small piece of crack). After spending minutes on the floor and finding nothing, she stormed into Nicco's room and discovered a fortune. Her eyes instantly grew bigger in size as she saw more cocaine than ever before laid across Nicco's bed. She paid no attention to the money, or the fact that Nicco was cussing her out like a dog. "What the fuck I tell you, 'bout busting into my room without knocking. All ya ass do is smoke and ain't never got no fucking money. Ya ass think Imma keep giving you shit? You got it fucked up. You better get out there and trick." Nicco said scolding his mother. "Now get the fuck out and next time knock first!" Nicco demanded. Still standing there with her eyes bulging out of their sockets, Joany only had one thing on her mind and that was kissing the sky! Jumping up off the bed, Nicco grabbed her by the arm and attempted to throw her out of the bedroom. To his surprise, she snatched away and backed hand the fuck out of him, as he stumbled back onto the bed looking stupid. "Nicholas Bartholomew Bob Johnson, don't you ever put your damn hands on me! The same way I bought you into this world, I'll take you the hell out of it, crack smoking or not!" Joany angrily stated. "Now give me something decent! Something that will hold me over for a couple of hours until I can get my hands on a few dollars." Joany pleaded. Looking at his mother like he wanted to give her ass some poison, he tossed a small zip lock bag at her that contained 1ounce. Catching the bag she said, "thank you baby", then hurried up out of the bedroom.

Back in the kitchen she wasted no time grabbing a pyrex and adding some water before placing it on top of the stove. Next she grabbed a box of baking soda and a butter knife then stood back at the stove and waited for the water to boil. Dropping the ounce of cocaine into the boiling water, Joany got greedy and decided to add the whole box of baking soda. Not knowing how pure the cocaine was, it could have easily ate two boxes of baking soda, to the one ounce tripling the weight. Shaking the pyrex in a slow circular motion she added a couple of ice cubes and continued the circular motion until a huge crack rock appeared. Happy as ever, she tried to remove the rock, but it was too big. Draining all the water out of the pyrex, she then took the butter knife and pressed down on the rock until it broke into two big pieces. Sitting back at the table she opened another can of 211, and started getting high. At first it seemed too good to be true! As she thought to herself, "All this crack and it's good! I have to get my hands on a few of them ounces. Little Nick will never know!" Exhaling thick white clouds of crack smoke. Joany drifted off into deep thought. "Shit if he gets locked up, I'll have full access to his supply. I can tell him somebody broke into the house, or that the cops came here with a search warrant and took everything they found. Or just maybe I can dip into his stash, and swap some of it out with a few packs of creatinine, he won't know the difference." Stuck from the effects of the crack, Joany sat there thinking all kind of devilish thoughts. Thinking about his next move, Nicco decided to call a nigga he knew from down 16th Street projects. Wasn't much going on over that part of Jersey city besides the bitches and a lil money. They both use to backdoor shit together years ago, but nowadays the nigga got on some other shit! He started running with these wild niggaz from out the Weequahic section in Newark! And all these niggaz do is shoot shit. If the price was right these niggaz will take the Presidents head off and be like fuck the time! These niggaz were savage beasts, but they respected All Made Men! "Nigga.what the fuck you been doing?" Keto asked as he answered the call. "Getting to that bag." Nicco replied. "I hear you fam, so what's good?" Keto asked. "You down for a job?" Nicco asked. "If the price is right." Keto answered. "I got a few bands for you and ya Goons. I need this bitch dead!" Nicco stated. "50rackz. Nothing less!" Keto stated. "Tell you what. I'll give the 50rackz, plus throw you a whole brick. Just get the job done!" Nicco stated. "Let me make sure I'm hearing this right?! Fifty Thousand and a whole chicken?" Keto asked. "All you!!" Nicco replied. "Who's the target?" Keto asked. "Some pretty bitch named Bliss!" Nicco stated. "Yo! You talking 'bout the nigga Kiem girl Bliss?" Keto asked. "Something like that!" Nicco said sarcastically. "You bugging B. I don't know about this one!" Keto said. "But I got some shooters in Brick City out in the Weequahic section. Same ticket though. You paying, or you playing?" Keto seriously asked. "Get with me tonight, I'll be parked on the corner of Bidwell and Jackson. You'll see my car soon as you hit the block. All money good!" Nicco said before hanging up. Thinking to himself why this nigga wanted Kiem's girl dead wasn't adding up! But the money and the whole chicken was, as Keto called one of his lil hitters from the Bricks. With the phone ringing for the seventh time, Bo$$ finally picked up! "What it do Keto?" Bo$$ asked. "Got some work lined up. You can rock dolo for a bigger portion, or you can split the pie." Keto said. You know my nigga gotta eat if I eat! We out this bitch together!" Bo$$ said. "What's the range?" "20rackz. all dirt time!" Keto stated. "My G! It's 30rackz a body, and that gotta get split two ways! So what you gonna do?" Bo$$ asked. "I got you lil nigga! Meet me in the back of my projects and two hours, and we move from there!" Keto stated. "Be there in a few!" Bo$$ said then hung up.

    With a few ounces bagged up and a couple of bricks in the North Face backpack, Nicco put the rest of the bricks back inside the army duffle bag and quietly carried it up to the attic. Stashing the duffle bag underneath some molded insulation, he checked that it was secure and quietly crept back downstairs. Still stuck at the table high as fuck, his moms never noticed him come past
her either time. Lifting his bed mattress up, he put an ounce and $200 underneath knowing that his moms would be in his room shortly searching for shit so this was the decoy to keep her at bay! Grabbing his car keys, he left out determined to be that nigga!

    Out the shower and fully dressed Kiem quickly started unloading his trunk with the laundry sacks full of cocaine. With everything except two laundry sacks upstairs in the bedroom, he carried the four sacks into the bathroom, where he then went to the bathtub and pressed down on the back edge of the tub and removed the whole thing! Once the tub was completely removed, he then entered the combination to the safe and expressed. "Well y'all already know, ain't no panties under these shorts! Besides that's some trife thot shit!" Bandz replied. "Speaking of panties, we gotta get you some clothes!" Kiem stated. "You feel like hitting the mall?" Kiem asked. "It's still time for you to snatch a few fits up. It's just now turning 7:45 pm." Don Smoke stated. "You gotta go dolo Bandz. We got work to do, and every second counts." Kiem explained. "Shiittt. I ain't got no worries mobbin' dolo!" Bandz stated. "I got you both on speed dial if I need ya! But this ain't what niggaz want and it damn sure ain't what bitches want!" Bliss said boldly as ever. "Factz." Kiem and Don Smoke both said. Reaching into the duffel bag, Kiem took out a stock of blue faces and handed it to Bandz. "This should hold you down, but make sure you get some all black everything!" Kiem stated. Staring into his eyes, she understood what Kiem was saying. "Oh before I forget! Here!!" Kiem opened the door panel on the entertainment center and gave her a chrome 380. "What da hell am I gone do with this pea shooter?" Bandz asked sarcastically. "Pop on instant!" Kiem replied. "No need to move with nothing big right now. At least you can conceal this in ya purse." Kiem stated. You right bein that I am half naked!" Bandz said laughing. "Let me breeze so I can get back! I know y'all hungry all that smokin' we been doin'. I'll grab some KFC or something!" Bandz said walking out the door. "My nigga! We got a lot of work to do. I'm gone need you to weigh out the baking soda while I whip! Once I turn twenty into sixty I'll have a good start. So you can go ahead and take the other hundred brickz and hit each one doubling the weight." Kiem explained. "We got our hands full, but we'll have enough ready to make shit shake! It's no way possible we'd be able to do everything in just one day but we'll get it done!" Kiem stated. "No question!" Don Smoke replied. Working four pots at one time, Kiem got down to business whipping the work while Don Smoke kept scaling the Arm & Hammer. With the air conditioner on and the air vents open you could still smell the potency of the cocaine in the air as it was being cooked up. Don Smoke looked on in amazement as Kiem dumped the first pot, then the second pot, the third, then the fourth! Four huge boulders of crack sat on top of the kitchen counter air drying. Don Smoke could easily eye each boulder, knowing that it weighed a little over 3,000 grams easy! A couple of hours had past and Kiem was already thirty-six brickz up. With only a few more left to whip before he reached his quota, he took a quick breather. As Bandz entered the den with all types of bags in her hands, smelling the chicken Kiem and Don Smoke looked on with disappointment in their eyes because they didn't see no type of bags that represented food. Opening an Ace Hardware bag, Bandz took out a 20-piece bucket of KFC, a 10 piece biscuits, and 3 cans of sprite. Fascinated by the food, Don Smoke and Kiem didn't hesitate to start crushing shit. The room was silent except for the licking of fingers, and the smacking from the chewing. Everyone sat in their own comfort zone and just ate while being nosy looking at each other. "Damn! Bandz eating like she been starving all her fucking life!" Don Smoke thought to himself. "Dis nigga here he needs to stop! Kiem u really looks pitiful eatin' like u ain't got no damn money". Bandz thought to herself. "Don Smoke you my nigga! But ya name should a been eat 'em ups! Slow down 'fore you choke 'cuz I don't know CPR. But I'll rush ya ass to the hospital!" Kiem thought to himself. All of a sudden everyone burst out laughing. "Whats so damn funny y'all?" Bandz asked. "I was hoping that you could tell us, being that ya ass was laughing too!" Kiem stated. "It was nothin'. Just a lil thought I had." Bandz replied. "Yea right! In that case, I guess we all had a lil thought." Don Smoke said laughing. "Thanks for the food Ma! A nigga was hungry as fuck! All that good weed a nigga had to eat something." Kiem stated. Throwing her legs up in the air and spreading 'em open. "U still hungry nigga?" Bandz asked sarcastically! "I'll pass!" Kiem stated then tossed a biscuit at her ass. "You do have a phat pussy!" Kiem said to himself as he went back in the kitchen and began whipping. Shaking his head Don Smoke got up and went into the kitchen and assembled the compressor. "My nigga! I'm gone slide on shit tonight. Just me and Bandz. We already got things lined up! After I finish tripling these eight brickz that will be exactly sixty already whipped up! Then I'm gone get suited and make sure everything's straight. With my calculations it should be no longer than a 5-6 hour trip. It's all about the speed, so we'll be back by sunrise! Come tomorrow we out and about getting back to that bag. When the news does travel everyone will be out in the clear." Kiem explained. "Say no more my nigga! I already know the count!" Don Smoke stated. "I'm 'bout to hit a few of these brickz, compress 'em, and wrap 'em. Any foul play hit me like yesterday! This ya call and I respect Bandz riding for the bro call." Don Smoke expressed. Dumping the last of the batch Kiem grinned as he stared at the 20 huge boulders laid across the kitchen countertop. Completing the 60 brickz of crack his work was almost done for the night. The only task left at hand was about to soon be executed as well. Saluting Don Smoke, Kiem looked him dead in the eyes then parted ways.

Heading upstairs to his bedroom he quickly stripped down and wiped off thoroughly with rubbing alcohol before putting his attire on. All black everything is how the scene takes place. From the boots, to the turtleneck, ski mask and gloves. Fully prepared and ready to slide, Kiem knocked on the next bedroom door as Bandz told him to enter. Her fitted jeans made her stand out like a cherry tree, but it was her black camouflage ski mask that caught Kiem's eye! The way that she was rocking it, reminded him of the street code "no face no case". "You ready?" Kiem asked. "Ready as can be!" Bandz replied. Tucking the 40 S&W inside its holster, she put on her jacket and zipped it close, concealing the weapon and its stick. After strapping on her backpack, she then grabbed Kiem by the hand and said "let's slide my G!" Bouncing downstairs to the garage, Kiem removed the tarp from the all Black Kawasaki Ninja. Handing Bandz a black helmet, he then put his own helmet on, then put on his gloves. Once he made sure Bandz helmet was secure, he got on the bike and started it up. Bandz quickly hopped on the back and held onto Kiem's waist. Looking back at her he told her to hold on, as he gassed the throttle. Nodding her head in agreement, Kiem hit the clutch and put the bike in first gear. Gliding out of the garage, Kiem hit the clutch and switched gears. as him and Bandz took off into the darkness of the night.

Sitting inside the late model MPV, Bo$$ waited for Keto to come downstairs so they can make moves. Shit was hot down here in his projects and sitting inside a mini van dirty wasn't making shit any better. No license, two guns, and open bottle of E&J, and some molly. Boy am I asking to go to jail?! Bo$$ thought to himself. "Oh shit!!" He said with excitement out loud while digging into his small upper jean pocket. Removing the folded bill he opened it up and smiled graciously. Reaching for the Newport box, he tore him querulous. $70,000 he quoted. "How the fuck I'm gonna pay $70,000 without the Feds snatching my black ass up?" He asked himself. Frustrated he got back in his and car drove off! Looking for a hotel, so he can relax for a couple days, the money had him wanting something extraordinary! Atlantic City was home to some of the best hotels on the East Coast! It had its reputation for hotels, casinos, the boardwalk, and the food! Live entertainment and I do mean live! Cuz right outside of the casino and down the street was the projects! And everything went down right outside! Turning into the Marriott, he parked and sat in deep thought about that HellCat! "I gotta get that whip!" He said out loud as he got out the car and walked into the lobby.

Making a sharp left on Dow Rd, Bandz leaned the bike with ease and proceeded to the house! Coming up the driveway the garage door instantly opened allowing quick entry to the garage. Turning the ignition off and removing their helmets, Kiem put them up on the shelf, then grabbed a few gallons of bleach. Laying two nylon tarps on the garage floor he told Bandz to stand in the middle and strip, as he stood beside her and did the same. Handing her a gallon of bleach, he told her to soak him from the neck down as he did her in return! Standing there in the nude, Bandz stated "Really nigga?! Bleach?!" Then asked. "What was da bleach for?" "To kill all DNA! Forensics can't get a match with shit being bleached down!" Kiem answered. Then they poured the remaining two gallons of bleach, all over the clothes they just had on soaking everything completely. Rolling the tarps up, then putting 'em inside of a doubled heavy duty black trash bag, Kiem tied the bag up, and sat it next to the garage door for trash pick up. "Ma! We gotta be quick and quiet for two reasons! 1.) Bro probably resting after being up all night doubling them brickz. 2.)We both ass naked. and I don't feel like explaining shit!" Kiem stated. "What da hell are you waitin' for?" Bandz asked as she made her way upstairs.

Hitting the shower soon as he got in the bedroom, he could hear Bandz doing the same in the master's bedroom next door. Standing under the shower head while the water rained down on him his thoughts began to flow! Thinking 'bout how deadly Bandz was, was a gift and a curse! A deadly gift for anybody that got out of pocket, and a curse upon herself if she didn't learn how to control her anger, which could end her career! Deep down inside he knew that Bandz was not to be played with, especially if you was an opp! But on the other hand, he knew that he had to show her everything that he was thinking, instead of just telling her! She reminded him so much of Bliss. Beautiful, intelligent, loyal, outspoken, deadly, and classy! Their style was so impeccable that they could of easily been someone's stylist, but she was part of the squad, and at the end of the day, she was good! No matter what the circumstances were.

Getting out of the shower. he wrapped a towel around his waist and exited the bathroom. Sitting on the edge of the bed, a gentle knock repeated at the door. "Yo!" Kiem called out. "Can I come in for a minute?" Bandz asked. "No doubt!" Kiem replied. Standing in a fuchsia robe she looked at Kiem and said. "I just wanna thank you for being real, loyal, and for always havin' my back! I never knew my father, and I never had a brother, so you da only male figure that I've ever known. Thankz for everything Kiem!" Bandz expressed. "You welcome Ma! You know I'm always gone do what's best for everybody! Loyalty is all I know!!!" Kiem replied. "But we will build more on things after we rest and get something to eat. Our line of work ain't finished, and we still have plenty of chips to get!" Kiem stated. "Say less!" Bandz stated then extended her arms to Kiem and gave him a hug before leaving the bedroom. Taking a deep breath. he laid back on the bed and sent Bliss a brief text! "I know it's early and your resting but always know that my loyalty is key! Key to unlock any door in these streetz or any lock within the universe! It's all about the journey and who you share it with! You are an amazing woman. Many women have done excellently, but you surpass them all. XO XO Kiem!"

Trying to put a scheme together, so he can pull off in that HellCat. Nothing was working for him! Everything he could possibly think of and everyone he could have thought of, was either a dead end, or they didn't fuck with him! So he had no choice but to reason with Karma in hopes of her being able to pull some kind of strings for him. Nicco hated the fact that he had to deal with this bitch once again! Knowing his plan was to jerk her for the money and the brickz off the rip! But being that he paid Keto to handle what he surely wasn't, it gave him a little leverage to manipulate Karma. Brainstorming about the bullshit he was gonna hit her with, he made a call to her at exactly 6:03am. Enjoying a fresh cup of Nantucket blend coffee, Karma sat in the nude at her bedroom breakfast table, preparing herself for the daily activities. Putting on an Azzedine Alaia, navy blue top and skirt, her phone began to ring, as she slipped on a pair of white Jimmy Choo heels. She allowed it to ring, taking her precious time because she already knew who it was. Getting annoyed from the constant phone ringing, she decided to answer, "Good morning darling! Is this phone call in reference to good news or business?" Karma asked. "Business." Nicco replied. "Good! Very good to know that you've been taking care of business and making the proper preparations to handle what's at large! I will meet with you shortly darling, but I must warn you, if anything is not what you say it to be, the streetz will know that you're a rat! Toodles darling!" Now stressing that the bitch just threatened him all he could do was figure out a way to get his way, then get far away! Nicco ain't give a fuck 'bout nothing if it wasn't concerning him. As long as he got his way, nothing else mattered!

The morning air was brisk, and the sky was cloudy and gray. It was one of them gloomy mornings that spoke to the streetz whenever somebody got killed! In Jersey City you could always feel it in the air whenever somebody got their wings clipped. Police had yellow taped the entire parking lot off, just a few feet from the playground, where the body of an unidentified man with two gunshot wounds to the head was found. Homicide was on the scene questioning a couple of joggers who always head out for an early morning run. Unsurprisingly, no one heard or saw a thing, and this type of shenanigan left homicide with nothing to go off of. With the coroners now on the scene, they immediately removed a stretcher from the back of the van along with a black body bag Placing the victim inside the bag, they quickly zipped it closed and put the body onto the stretcher then strapped it down before hauling it off. On his way back from East Orange, Nice took Communipaw Ave all the way up and saw police everywhere as he drove past Lincoln Park. Observing the scene, he noticed that homicide was out there, as well as the coroner, with the news van arriving up on the scene. "What the fuck happened out here?" He questioned himself as he continued driving. Knowing that he was dirty, he kept it

Relaxed and high like a kite Don Smoke headed into the kitchen and got situated with the tag and bag process. Taking 10 of the boulders that Kiem had whipped up, he began busting 'em down, as Bandz walked into the kitchen with a metric scale in her hand. Weighing each boulder out that was broke down, at a lil over 1,000 grams a piece. Bandz took a sharpie and tagged each zip lock with its exact weight, then bagged it. Two hours had gone by since the process began, and the results were 30 brickz easy! Taking 15 of the brickz that was already tagged and bagged, Bandz stuffed them into a small size gym bag then placed the other 15 inside of an ottoman in the den. Down in the garage, Don Smoke's phone started ringing while he was in the process of stashing 20 brickz, inside his car floor compartment. After closing the compartment, he called the number back and discussed locations. With everything ready that was set to be moved, Bandz grabbed her gun up off of the garage counter and held it by her waistline. Once she got inside the Audi she placed her girlfriend in her lap, then twist a backwood. Riding dirty was nothing to either one of them, the routine was so consistent that it became a norm. In route to the first drop off, Don Smoke cut the AC on, and cracked the panoramic roof while Bandz fired up! Arriving at the address on N St NW, Kiem turned up into the Iron Gate parking lot and backed into a parking space. Entering the restaurant he scanned the entire place looking unnoticeable, as he spotted his connect sitting at an end table section, with a light skin woman wearing a Dark Grey pants suit. As Kiem approached the table, Oscar stood to his feet and shook hands while greeting him. "Glad that you could join me, my friend!" Oscar stated. No problemo!" Kiem replied. "Ahh my friend! You've been sharpening your espanol!" Oscar said pleased. "Please have a seat!" Oscar said calmly as he introduced the woman sitting next to him. "This here is FBI special agent, Ms. Kym Guy." "Nice to meet you sir!" She greeted while extending her hand. Looking on in disgust he couldn't believe that he was sitting in the presence of a federal agent. Not knowing what the fuck was next, Kiem pulled his Glock and aimed at the agent's head! Quickly rising to his feet, Oscar put his hand in front of the gun and pushed it away from the agent's head, before saying. "My friend she's one of us!" "How the fuck she's one of us, and she's the fucking Feds?" Kiem angrily asked. "I do most sincerely apologize for not raising your awareness!" Oscar stated. "However, my good friend, she works for me. Which means she works for us! I've employed Ms. Guy for over two decades now and have been extremely successful in all of my undertakings!" Oscar expressed. "She's here on business to inform you about a foe you've done business with." Oscar stated. "It seems that you have a leak that needs to be plugged immediately!" "Sir, if you will allow me a few minutes of your time this whole situation can be clear before it gets too late!" Kym stated. Placing a brief case on top of the table, she opened it and slid several pictures of Nicco across the table to Kiem. "I take it that you know this person?" She asked. "Why? What's up?" Kiem impatiently answered the question with a question. "He was arrested on a bullshit traffic stop and while he was being taken into custody. Jersey City's finest searched his vehicle and found 3 kilos of cocaine. He instantly cooperated with authorities for a free pass and gave a full statement! Here's all the copies of his written statement, along with several pictures of him inside of the surveillance room being interviewed, while giving a written statement! The case was somehow swept under the rug and never made it to even be processed for my department to indict him on Federal charges. But this is where things get tricky. A Lieutenant down at the 5th precinct in Jersey City managed to get hold of the paperwork and fax everything over to my Captain. My partner, Jeff Hoilday and I, are now assigned to the case! He's being indicted on federal charges for possession of 3 kilos of cocaine. My partner's a real prick and he's looking for some type of glory so that he can move up in rank. Now here's the thing! He's going to cooperate with the prosecutors which means. he gets little to no time at all, while the federal grand jury gets a conviction. And if you're convicted, you're looking at least 200 - 250 months minimum, which is between 20 - 25 years. I would advise you to secure your freedom by any means necessary! Do not worry about my partner. I will take of him!" Kym said in a cold but serious tone of voice. Thankful for catching this wave, Kiem sat in silence for a moment thinking about the time when he served Nicco 3 brickz, and how Ms. Estelvo pulled up on him out of nowhere! Was it all a setup? Using Nicco, to get to me? He questioned himself. But why would this bitch want to get close to me? What is it that she wants from me? Kiem continued questioning himself. Snapping out of his zone he calmly stated, "Whatever is necessary will be taken care of on my end! You need to make sure that your end is taken care of as well!" Sharply nodding her head in agreement, FBI special agent Kym Guy excused herself from the table. As she stood and headed in the direction of the ladies' room, Kiem and Oscar both witnessed that she had urinated on herself. Quickly locking the door behind her, she leaned her back up against it, as she took a few deep breaths trying to regain her composure! Removing her pants and then her panties she tossed her panties into the trashcan, then took a few sanitary napkins and wiped herself thoroughly. Using the hand soap, she instantly cleaned her pants where it was needed then held them up underneath the hand dryer to quickly dry. Looking into the mirror, she wanted to break down and cry, knowing that she was almost a dead bitch! But she understood Kiem's point of view, not knowing her line of work, or who she was. Quickly putting her pants back on, she washed her hands, then headed back to the table. "Welcome back!" Oscar stated. Embarrassed by not knowing if either one of them noticed her accident, she looked away in shame! "Shall we eat now?" Oscar asked striving to break the silence. Kiem was in his own world plus rolling off the Molly so everything was enhanced. He felt no type of way about pulling out on the federal agent. After all, she was still a federal agent, regardless to what his connect said. Even if she did make good on her end, she was still the Feds and Kiem didn't fuck with twelve in no shape, form, or fashion! But utilizing her resources was only as good as he allowed. Kiem was sharp. He saw the good cop, bad cop role before, so when it came to the streetz. he could advance on any level. Time was moving as a waitress wheeled a serving cart over to the table with a desired dish for prepared for everyone. Kiem and his connect enjoyed Roasted-Lobster Bucatini, while the federal agent enjoyed a warm Shrimp Salad. Breaking his silence, Kiem said to federal agent, "I want you to know that it was business, nothing personal." Looking him dead in the eyes, she replied, "I can understand your logic, I probably would have done the same." "My friend! Time moves rapidly when you're enjoying good food huh!" Oscar stated. "Ms. Kym Guy! Please allow me to honor our business! For any discomfort that may have been caused, I give to you 100k.

right signal light on Don Smoke turned into the Hampton Inn parking lot, as Kiem hit his high beams twice, then kept it moving. Knowing that his nigga was good him and Bandz headed back to the house! "I fuckz with da Porsche!" Bandz stated. "But you my nigga for real Kiem! I ain't gone lie, if I could have you trust, it would be just that! But I like flirting with you, you don't let that shit go to ya head! Most of da time, I just enjoy being in ya presence. Besidez wheneva we out and 'bout, we married nigga! My loyalty to is to you and to protect you as well nigga!" Bandz expressed. "Ya doing a great job Ma! Keep up the good work!" Kiem stated. "But we're gonna further discuss things when we get to the house. We have a lot of work to take care of, plus I need to check some shit! But for right now. I want you to relax and let ya thoughts flow! Figure out what it is that you want out of life, and how you gonna get it! Most importantly I want you to take time to understand ya self, get to know who you are! I want you to know ya worth and value it. Strengthen all ya weak points and understand ya power!" Kiem sincerely expressed. Mesmerized by what Kiem just told her, Bandz positioned herself in the passenger's seat in a relaxed posture, then reached for Kiem's right hand and held it tightly. Looking at her, Kiem knew that he just penetrated her mental. Focusing his eyes back on the road, he pushed the Porsche with ease back to New Castle.

Turning his headlights off Nicco entered the main disposal dump site and drove up to the feed conveyor belt. The machine was operating, and the belt was moving rapidly feeding whatever laid on it, into the huge dump disposal. Looking around nervously, Nicco didn't see anybody! He already knew that he had to do whatever it takes to dispose of his mother's remains. Quietly getting out of his car, he opened the trunk and reached for the rug. Struggling to lift it up, he paused for a second, then he was able to grab a firmer hold of it the second time around. Carrying the rug over to the machine, he threw it onto the feed belt and watched as his mother's remains, went up the belt and into the main dump disposal. Once the rug was out of clear view, he quickly got into his car and drove off! Confused with everything that just happened Nicco couldn't understand the message that was being sent! Now trying to figure out where he was gonna tuck his tail at for the night was the impossible. Wanting to call Cheebah was his first thought but knowing that Shark could come through at any time wasn't a bright idea. He thought about calling Keto but wasn't sure if he had taken care of things, and if so, that was out the question too! Turning his headlights back on, paranoia started to kick in. Looking in his rearview nonstop he almost ran a red light. Looking in every direction as he drove, one would think that he was on Angel Dust the way he was tripping out! Knowing that he couldn't go back to the house, his only thought was to burn the bitch to the ground. But doing it himself wasn't gonna happen. He knew that he couldn't just up and disappear without raising anyone's suspicion either, so he had to figure something out quickly! "Maybe I can get Keto, or the young nigga who runs with him, to take care of this shit! It ain't nothing but an arson job. Five thousand should be more than enough to get it done." Nicco said out loud to himself. Searching for a lowkey spot, Nicco decided to get a room at The Double Tree. I'll just post up here for the next few days, then head south after my party he thought to himself.

Backing into the garage, Bandz was knocked out while still holding a tight grip on Kiem's hand. "Ma! Get up!" He said while shaking her arm with his hand still held in hers. "Daammmnnn nigga! U tryna break my arm?" Bandz angrily asked startled out of her sleep. Looking at her in disbelief he didn't even respond, knowing that he had startled her. "Wait right here for a minute!" Kiem stated then got out of the car and walked around to his passenger's side. He opened the door and scooped Bandz up into his arms. "Feel better now?" He asked sarcastically as he carried her into the house. "A lil bit but my arm hurts! You tried to pull my arm out of socket boy!" Bandz replied sad fully fucking with Kiem. Laughing at her response, he turned away from her, took two steps then instantly fell out. Quickly rushing to his aide, she started pulling on him, and screaming his name. "Kiem! Kiem!" Opening his eyes he looked at her, then said "I thought ya arm hurts!" Punchin' him in the chest, Bandz was pissed! She punched him again then said "Nigga! Don't you ever play with me like that again!" Grabbing him by his shirt collar she then stated. "I'm serious nigga!" "You got it Ma! But we even now!" Kiem stated in a playful tone of voice. "Even my ass nigga! You heard what I said!" Bandz said seriously. Getting up from the floor, Kiem pulled her close to him and gave her a hug. "Ma. Listen! I told you that you got it. I can understand your anger so it won't happen again!" Kiem stated. "You mutha fuckin right it won't!" Bandz said still feeling some type of way. "But I forgive you nigga! You know I got to take ya ass through da ringer!" Bandz stated. "Check though! You was right about Nicco's bitch ass being a rat! My connect got 12 on the payroll, I'm talkin' FBI. The nigga got caught with 3 brickz. Brickz that I sold him. So when he got bagged for a bullshit traffic stop, 12 searched his car and found the work. The nigga gave a statement and exchange for walking papers. I seen the paperwork. Pictures of him in the surveillance room being interviewed and all types of shit. The fed that works for my connect, is now assigned to the case along with her partner. She said that her partner is a real dick head, looking to pull rank! Nicco is about to get indicted on federal charges for possession of 3 kilos of cocaine. Now he gets little or no time at all for his cooperation. They build a case on me, he cooperates, I go to federal prison. The FBI partner makes captain. She told me to secure my freedom, and not to worry 'bout her partner! Bottom line, without a witness, they don't have a case! But the puzzle is still incomplete cuz what I do know is, Ms. Estelvo been in on this whole ordeal from the jump! She pulled up on me out of nowhere one day, the same day that I sold Nicco the work. The bitch might've been in the cut somewhere, just watching the whole time. Cuz it's impossible, that she just gone come from outta nowhere. At that exact location at that! Question is what is it that she wants from me." "Kiem. This shit is like some kinda fatal attraction, stalker type shit!" Bandz said in a concerned tone of voice. "But we gone slide on Nicco's rat azz!" She then stated with a voice full of hostility. "That bitch made nigga, gone suffer for this one! But the chapter ain't done 'til we close the book!" Bandz stated in a calm but sinister tone of voice.

Enjoying each other's company. Don Smoke and Kola shared some interesting conversations, over a few shots of Ketel One Grapefruit & Rose Vodka. Kola even went to the extreme and popped a piece of Molly with Don Smoke! It was her first time taking any type of drug. She started to get loose and feel relaxed. Still in her right state of mind, small neither. She had a stripper type body and a little cuteness to go with it, but anyone could tell that she was on one due to the constant sniffles. Still she was what someone would call, " a nice time!" Shaking her ass to French Montana's Unforgettable had Bo$$ ready to beat something! Enjoying the live entertainment, he never realized that he had a missed call. He quickly dialed the number back. "Holla!" Nicco stated as he answered his phone. "Yo! I just seen that I had a missed call from this number." Bo$$ said. "Who this?" Nicco asked. "You called my phone b and you got the nerve to be questioning who am I." Bo$$ stated in an aggressive tone of voice. "My nigga Keto wifey gave me your number, and the message from him! So you trying to get that bag or what?" Nicco said. "Am I." Bo$$ replied. "The names Bo$$, I'm Keto's lil hitman!" He stated. "I was hoping this number was your number, 'cuz I'm trying to discuss some real business with you!" Nicco said like he was some type of shot caller for real. "State your claim big man!" Bo$$ said in hopes of stroking Nicco's ego. "I need you to set some shit a blaze for me, and I have this bitch that Keto and you was supposed to take care of before he got bagged!" "I can dig it! Bo$$ replied. "But here's the thing. I need my money upfront! I don't do that cash on delivery shit!" Bo$$ stated. "How much you talking?" Nicco asked. "Thirty grand for the bitch and five grand for the arson!" Bo$$ stated. "I tell you what how 'bout I throw you a whole chicken for everything! That's the price you're asking, plus extra!" Nicco stated. "You mean to tell me you gonna give me a whole thang to handle this shit for you?" Bo$$ asked. "The whole thang." Nicco replied. "Where do we meet?" Bo$$ asked. "Are you familiar with Jersey City?" Nicco asked. "Not for real!" Bo$$ replied. "Can you meet me on Broad St. in about 45 mins?" Nicco asked. "Sure thing! I can make it there sooner if you need me to." Bo$$ replied. "Nah! 45 mins is good." Nicco said. "Also you know where I can get a hammer from?" "Depends on my what you looking for?" Bo$$ replied. "Just a handgun or something for now!" Nicco stated. "Let me see what I can come up with and I'll get with you when we meet." Bo$$ stated. "That'll work!" Nicco replied. "What you driving so I'll know your car when I pull up?" Bo$$ asked. "Imma be two cars deep playa soon as I get there I will hit your phone!" Nicco said in arrogant tone. "I'm about to be on my way!" Bo$$ replied. "I'll catch you then!" Nicco stated then hung up. Thinking too himself that was probably the most smartest thing he'd ever done in his life. Telling some nigga he just agreed to business with, that he don't even know, that he'll be riding two cars deep! Nicco knew how shiesty niggaz could be cuz the same shit flowed through his veins! Not to mention that he inquired about purchasing a handgun. Making an appointment to drop off a whole brick without a gun is a straight sign of "I'm 'bout to jack this nigga!" Pulling the duffle bag out from underneath the bed, he opened it and took out a brick then took out 3 stackz of blue faces. Tearing the band off one of the stackz, he counted out a thousand then put it inside of his pocket. Grabbing the white plastic ice bag from the hotel room table, he put the brick inside of it, then stuffed the rest of the money into his jacket pocket and made ways to go meet the young nigga Bo$$.

Happy as ever that his finesse just got him paid, and he didn't have to shoot a nigga was sweet money for him! Thinking about how he could've taken a chance and robbed the nigga, probably would've got him laid out knowing that the nigga was riding two cars deep. Instead he just got paid to do what he do, for the second time! Bo$$ told shorty to throw some clothes on and ride with him right quick! "We need to make this appointment on time. We handled the hard part already, now it's a cakewalk!" Bo$$ said in greedy tone of voice. "Bring ya ass shorty!" He yelled out at her. "I'm coming damn! You wanna rush somebody, and I'm the one that made the nigga believe the bullshit!" She said sounding irritated. "Just bring ya ass! You'll thank me later!" Bo$$ said.

With all the money counted, Don Smoke was witnessing Kiem's vision live and direct. A few more rounds like this and we'll be able to network the whole East Coast. He thought to himself. And being that he had met Kola, time would only tell if she was worth it! But Don Smoke had a vision and just like Kiem, his vision was for the squad! Bandz did her thing handling the tag and bag. Sitting at the table Don Smoke twisted a backwood, while him and Bandz talked about how crazy the money was coming in. With the RPK in the air Kiem came downstairs into the kitchen and dapped Don Smoke up, before giving Bandz a hug. "Hey sleepy head!" Bandz said to Kiem. "Never sleepy Ma! Tired as fuck. Sleep is the cousin of death! Always remember that!" Kiem said to her. "I gotcha my nigga!" She replied. "So you enjoy ya self my nigga?" Kiem asked Don Smoke. "You already know the count my nigga!" Don Smoke said smiling. "Yo! She a high profile lawyer out here! She owns her own firm, plus she owns another firm out in Cali!" He stated. "That's what's up my nigga! She's a money maker!" Kiem said. "Yea! Plus all her friends that she was with all professionals! Lawyers, Gynecologists, and Head Prosecutors!" Don Smoke explained. "They doing their thing!" Kiem stated in approval. "We moving on shit tomorrow night! After I finish Nicco's ass, we shootin' out to Connecticut! We gone run through Hammer Time and smash everything! Once we hit that safe and lay everything! We gone blow back out here and post up, 'til we ready to hit Maryland and North Carolina! We got product on the agenda for Va., but once I contact a few of my niggaz out there, we let them move the weight! That foreign bitch picked the wrong poison this time!" Kiem expressed in a hostile but relaxed manner. Heading to the back room, he retrieved the guns, the extra extensions and the hook knife that he removed from the safe. Making his way back to the kitchen he sat all the artillery on the table. "Nigga it's definitely on and poppin'!" Bandz stated as she grabbed the Tec and cocked it. Don Smoke already knew that the Mac was for him when he viewed it. It was more his style when it came to semi's, unless it was an AK. "What's the knife for?" Bandz asked. "You ever seen a rat get its guts ripped out then ate by some wolves?" Kiem asked Bandz. "Nigga you buggin' out. Ya ass sound like you could be the Black Stephen King," Laughing at her comment Kiem continued. "Bandz, Nicco is gone be down on you once he sees you! Make it hard for him but lead him to think that you want him! I'm gone need for you to lure him into Steak City Warehouse downtown. Then you just sit back and enjoy the show!" Kiem said in a cold tone of voice. "Don Smoke I'm gone need you close by to keep an eye out on the streetz! Once I handle this we bounce straight to Connecticut and eat! This is the key! Leave room for no mice!" Kiem stated seriously. "Bandz you gone have to get XL or one of the Sexes to take ya G-Wagon back to ya spot after the club. Everything is all about the timing!" Kiem explained. "That's no problem. XL will take care of that for sure!" Bandz said. "Don Smoke take the four duffle bags in the with you to see a doctor and to keep you company while I'm taking care of things." He explained. "No bae! I'm good!" She replied. "You're not! So this is not even up for discussion!" He said. Bliss threw the towel in. "Alright! I'll go and she can keep me company." Bliss replied. "Great! I'll have her get with you tomorrow and the two of you can arrange things." "Bliss I have to make some runs then I'll be back! I'll bring you some food so you won't have to worry 'bout cooking later." "That's fine bae!" She replied then thanked him for always making sure that she was good. "You don't have to thank me Ma! It's my responsibility to make sure that you good." He replied. Giving her a peck on the lips he whispered. "I'll be back!" then went on about his business.

Don Smoke just left the barbershop and heard something similar to what Shark had told his barber. The context was the same just worded different. Knowing that if he just caught wave, Kiem definitely caught wave, so it was no need to hit his phone! In route to pick up one of his shipments he knew the weed was exotic! His Cali connect stayed with shit a nigga couldn't even pronounce which made the value of the bud increase. Not only did he have fire on deck, he also kept some pure grade Molly which made Don Smoke untouchable on the East Coast.

Stopping at a Home Depot in Hoboken, Kiem went inside and purchased two Tyvek suits along with a 50 pack of zip ties. After the purchase, he hit a low key barbershop in the Spanish section of Hoboken. Out of sight, out of mind. Getting a low cut Cesar with the grain, his waves stood out even more than they did when he had a full head of hair. Checking out his cut in the mirror, the barber brushed him off, then removed the smock. Giving the barber a hundred-dollar bill, Kiem nodded his head at him, then continued with his runs. Making his final stop at a Jersey Mike's, he went inside and ordered him and Bliss a honey roasted Turkey sandwich, with provolone cheese, lettuce, tomatoes, oil, salt, pepper, and vinegar, two sprites, and two bags of kettle cooked plain potato chips. He then made his way back home. Once there he headed upstairs and entered the bedroom, noticing Bliss was not around. Hearing the shower water run, he knew that she must've been showering! Sitting on the bed along with the food, he unwrapped his sandwich and started to eat. Bliss entered the bedroom naked, as her long wavy wet hair, draped down her backside. Looking Kiem in the eyes, as she bent over putting coconut oil on her legs and all over her body made Kiem want to eat her instead of the sandwich. Bliss knew what she was doing, and Kiem knew it too but he enjoyed the mini thrill of watching her oil her body down, as he crunched on the chips and the sandwich. "Ooh! Jersey Mike's! My favorite! Thank you bae!" Bliss said then gave Kiem a kiss. "Fresh cut. You look good!" She stated. "Thankz!" He replied. Throwing on Kiem's Giants jersey, she sat down on the bed and began to eat. "How you feeling?" Kiem asked. Talking with a mouth full of food she managed to say alright. "Swallow ya food first then talk!" She laughed then said, "I'm alright for now but I still feel sluggish and sometimes dizzy. But I'm gonna get some rest after I eat, and if I still feel like this in the morning, I'm definitely going to the doctor." "Yea! You might have a stomach virus or something!" He replied. Finishing his sandwich and chips he downed the sprite like he was dying of thirst. Going into the closet, he looked through his designer before he grabbed the gray leather short sleeve Ferragamo pants suit and a pair of gray leather

Bally's. Taking a quick shower, Kiem had to get a move on things. Main Event was a thriller. It was the only club that jumped at 10:00 pm on. Out the shower and ready to get dressed, Bliss stepped up and oiled Kiem's body down! Wanting to tease him with her tongue she knew it was best to wait being that he had business to take care of. Throwing on a pair of Human Made boxer briefs and t-shirt, he followed up with the socks, then got fully dressed. Putting on both of his chains, made Bliss say "Bae you need a scarf the way ya neck is on freeze! You gone get sick going outside like that!" As they both laughed. Once he put the Daytona on Bliss instantly caught feelings! She didn't say nothing, but Kiem read her facial expression followed by her body language. Grabbing his Glock he put a thirty stick in it, cocked it, then tucked it in his waistline. Reaching in his pants pockets from the day before he removed the money that he had won from the casino. Handing Bliss $10k. She asked "What's this for?" "I want you to have half of my winnings." He said. "Ya winnings?" She questioned. "Yea! I hit the casino and won $70k." He replied. "So how's this half?" She questioned. "I split the money with Don and Bandz too!" He replied. "This is why you're perfect for me and I love you unconditionally! You always make sure that you take care of ya niggaz and show them the same loyalty and love that they show you!" She said with all sincerity. She kissed him and held him tightly. They let go of each other and headed towards the garage so Kiem could be on his way. "Wow! This is really all you right here." Bliss said soon as she laid eyes on the 4 door Porsche. "You like it?" He asked. "Hell yea! I love it!" She replied. "Look I gotta get going. I'm gonna send for everybody sooner than later. We all gone take a lil break, and just enjoy some time with each other." He expressed. Once the garage door opened the Panamera took off swiftly, as Bliss stood there smiling. Talking through his Bluetooth phone car system, Kiem let Don Smoke know that he'd be pulling up shortly. The 7 Sexes was already there and Rose XL did exactly what she said she was going to do! "Stop everything moving!" Her ass wiggled something seriously every time she took a step. The Sexes all had on different color cat suits! But Bandz took the cake with her white floral lace cat suit, fuchsia pink G-string, and a pair of all white red bottoms. She stood out the most from any other female up in the club. Her hair style was enough to make any bitch envy her. She had a Toni Braxton cut dyed fuchsia pink with three fine parts across her right backside neckline. Her Gold neck choker said "Pink Bandz" with enough diamonds that her name could easily be read from a distance! Don Smoke stood doing his normal, watching everything that moves. When an all Red HellCat pulled into the parking lot, playing Fat Joe's All the way up, everyone paid close attention to see who was pushing the whip. Nicco stepped out with his lil chain and shit on! Immediately, Don Smoke wanted to snatch this niggaz soul from him, but he knew that he had to be humble and play the role of a fool. The HellCat was tight though. Don thought to himself. But that type of money for a Dodge wasn't flyin' with him!

The parking lot was lit. Everybody was out there doing their thing before entering the club. Gi-Gi, was looking right in her Black silk cat suit. She had a body that niggaz craved, but barely showed it. Nevertheless, she could give a damn 'bout a nigga chasing her if it wasn't someone whom she'd desired as well. From a distance you could hear French Montana's song A lie blasting through someone's car system! Everyone in the

the R8 in gear and took off! Bandz looked on anxiously not knowing what the fuck was happening, as she heard multiple shots fired! Suddenly Kiem came dashing out of the door and made it to his car. Jumping inside he quickly grabbed the AR and let that bitch bang out the panoramic roof top! Cakk. Cakk. Cakk.Cakk. Cakk. Cakk. Cakk. Cakk. Cakk. Cakk. Kiem laid out everything that exited the door. Bandz pulled off doing 0-70 quick! Shots were fired back but nothing hit the Silver Beauty, as Bandz pushed the Porsche precisely. Making good time while moving with the darkness of the night, Bandz suddenly had a moment! "Woooooo!" She yelled out loud! She never felt such an adrenaline rush. Looking at her 'cuz he knew the feeling, Kiem sat in silence and allowed her to enjoy her moment. Pushing the Panamera. Bandz had all type of business ideas running through her head, knowing that Kiem was the reason behind her being so focused and determined. He had bought out the best in her! Kiem was well grounded when it came to handling business, and he instilled the same knowledge and discipline within everyone he came in contact with. The squad was all the way up now and Kiem knew that Ms. Estelvo would come for his head. But it was just a matter of her ignorance, versus his intelligence! Rule number 1. you can't go to war broke. Rule number 2. always keep ya opponents off balance! Rule number 3. always remember, dead men tell no toles!

     After about 25 minutes they reached their destination. Throwing the Porsche in park, Bandz and Kiem got out of the car, and made their way up into the den. Don Smoke had all four duffle bagz placed on the floor next to each other while burning a backwood. Passing the backwood to Kiem, Kiem took a deep long pull, then picked up one of the duffle bagz and emptied it out on the floor! "Let's count this fuckin' money!" He said to Don Smoke and Bandz. Dumping the bagz onto the floor, Bandz and Don Smoke went to work. A few hours had passed by and the count was at 37 million, with stackz and stackz still left to count! They couldn't believe that they just pulled off the biggest caper ever. By 9 am, the count ended at fifty million! The question now was how to invest the money without the Feds getting onto their ass! Don Smoke said. "I have an idea! I can holla at someone that has a friend who's a financial advisor. We all can gain some important advice and make wiser decisions from there!" "I'm with you my nigga!" Kiem said. "Yea! Me too!" Bandz said while fanning herself with a few stackz of blue faces." This what it is! Kiem stated. We divide the money at 16.5 a piece, and the last 500k, we invest it into something that can benefit everyone! From here on out we let our money talk for us! We don't get our handz dirty, unless we have too! All photographers on deck! I'm gone schedule to meet with the connect, we 'bout to buy into his network. But for the most part stay on point! That bitch is definitely gonna try to come for the kid, and it's no telling who she might target to try and get to me! She doesn't know nothing 'bout The Sexes which is good! Don you my nigga so she might target you, knowing that we rock like that." Kiem explained. We bang out. 'til we can't bang no more! That bitch power is only as good as her intelligence! And she's a dumb bitch. We also have to hit a few states that we normally do business in. This will give us time to let the heat die down as we move this work! But don't get too comfortable! Until I can make a move and finish Ms. Estelvo as of right now we work 24/7." Kiem explained. Bandz and Don Smoke, knew what Kiem was saying, and they understood what it was that had to be done for them to be successful. "Yo! I'm 'bout to hit The Breakfast Café. Anybody want anything?" Kiem asked. "Yea! You know what I want my nigga! Some scrambled eggs with cheese, grits, turkey sausage, and corned beef hash! And a few slices of wheat toast!" Don Smoke stated. "Damnnn u greedy!" Bandz said sarcastically. "I gotta feed the dick!" Don Smoke replied laughing. "What da fuck ever!" Bandz said. "I'm riding with you Kiem." "Let's bounce then! Be back shortly my nigg!" Kiem stated. Tucking her Glock, they went downstairs into the garage hopped in the Porsche and went on their way to get some breakfast. It was just 20 mins past 9:00 am., and the morning air was crisp and dry! Pulling up in front of The Breakfast Café a group of niggaz was posted up on the corner, doing whatever it was that they was out there doing, while looking at Kiem's car, with admiration in their eyes! Kiem's phone started to ring, as he put the Porsche in park! Looking at his caller ID, he'd noticed that it was a 757 area code number calling. It's gotta be one of my Va. niggaz not too many people have this number! He thought to himself. Answering the call an automated voice system announced. "You have a prepaid call from Quando! Press 1 to accept the call, 2 to deny the call, or 3 to block the party calling!" Pressing 1 with the quickness, Kiem listened to his young nigga excitedly talk! "What's good my nigga? I wanted to hit you up sooner, but I just been on my workout shit, getting closer to the door!" His young nigga stated. "That'z what it do my G! How you holding up in there?" Kiem asked. "You know the count bruh. Same old shit, just a different day! But I need a few dollars to hold me down ' til I reach the door!" Quando explained. "Say less my G!" "Kiem I'm getting hungry!" Bandz stated cutting his conversation off! "Yo! Hold on a minute!" Kiem told his young nigga over the phone. "Bandz order me the same thing that you get Don with two kiwi waters! I already know you gone get some shit! The food is off the chain here!" Kiem said then gave Bandz two blue faces! Looking at him puzzled she then asked "Two hundred dollars for some breakfast?" "I always tip 'em. Besides ain't shit cheap in there!" Kiem explained. before getting back to his conversation. "My bad my nigga! I had to order some food right quick!" Kiem stated. "You good bruh! Trust me! I know how that shit be, when you hungry!" Quando expressed. Ya information still the same? Kiem asked! "Already!" Quando replied. Look.I'm 'bout to Jpay you $300 right now, and I'm gone put $200 on ya phone account! Kiem explained. "Oh! You really doing big things my nigga!" Quando stated. "Gotta make sure all my niggaz are good! We all a team no matter the situation!" Kiem said. "All the time!" Quando replied. Look. when you get home, I'm gone get you situated! I don't want you out there fuckin' with nobody, that don't have ya best interest at heart! A lot of niggaz be fakin', but it's all on you to see thing's for what they are, rather than what they appear to be! Kiem explained. "Bruh. I understand where you coming from! You always dropping some deep shit on a nigga!" Quando replied.

Watching Bandz exit the restaurant, one of the niggaz posted outside approached her. "What's up nigga?" Bandz asked with a voice full of hostility. "I means no harm. I was just hoping that I can get your name and maybe your number! You're beautiful and I'm not gonna lie, your ass is like wow!! The names Honcho!" He expressed. "I'm Bandz but I'm kinda in a hurry!" "Fuck that bitch Honcho!" One of the niggaz standing on the corner yelled out! "Ya mommaz a bitch and ya faggot ass daddy's a bitch!" Bandz fired

THE MAN IN THE HIGH-WATER BOOTS

By F. Hopkinson Smith

1909

Now and then in my various prowlings I have met a man with a personality; one with mental equipment, heart endowment, self-forgetfulness, and charm—the kind of charm that makes you glad when he comes and sorry when he goes.

One was a big-chested, straight-backed, clear-eyed, clean-souled sea-dog, with arms of hickory, fingers of steel, and a brain in instant touch with a button marked "Experience and Pluck." Another was a devil-may-care, barefooted Venetian, who wore a Leporello hat canted over one eye and a scarlet sash about his thin, shapely waist, and whose corn teeth gleamed and flashed as he twisted his mustache or threw kisses to the pretty bead-stringers crossing Ponte Lungo. Still a third was a little sawed-off, freckled-faced, red-headed Irishman, who drove a cab through London fogs in winter, poled my punt among the lily-pads in summer, and hung wall-paper between times.

These I knew and *loved*; even now the cockles of my heart warm up when I think of them. Others I knew and *liked*; the difference being simply one of personality.

This time it is a painter who crosses my path—a mere lad of thirty two or three, all boy-heart, head, and brush. I had caught a glimpse of him in New York, when he "blew in" (no other phrase expresses his movement) where his pictures were being hung, and again in Philadelphia when some crushed ice and a mixture made it pleasant for everybody, but I had never examined all four sides of him until last summer.

We were at Dives at the time, lunching in the open courtyard of the inn, three of us, when the talk drifted toward the young painter, his life at his old mill near Eure and his successes at the Salon and elsewhere. Our host, the Sculptor, had come would be just as well, once in a while, to slip the tape around their chests and waists. Steam is what makes the wheels go round, and steam is well-digested fuel and a place to put it. With this equipment a man can put "GO" into his business, strength into his literature, virility into his brush; without it he may succeed in selling spool cotton or bobbins, may write pink poems for the multitude and cover wooden panels with cardinals and ladies of high degree; in real satin and life-like lace, but no part of his output will take a full man's breath away.

Sunshine, flowers, open windows letting in the cool breezes from meadow and stream; an old beamed ceiling, smoke-browned by countless pipes; walls covered with sketches of every nook and corner about us; a table for four, heaped with melons, grapes, cheese, and flanked by ten-pin bottles just out of the brook; good-fellowship, harmony of ideas, courage of convictions—with no heads swelled to an unnatural size; four appetites—enormous, prodigious appetites; Knight for host and Marie as high chamberlainess, make the feast of Lucullus and the afternoon teas of Cleopatra but so many quick lunches served in the rush hour of a downtown restaurant! Not only were the trout-baked-in cream (Marie's specialty) all that the Sculptor had claimed for them, but the fried chicken, soufflés—everything, in fact, that the dear woman served— would have gained a Blue Ribbon had she filled the plate of any committeeman making the award.

With the coffee and cigars (cigarettes had been smoked with every course—it was that kind of a feast) the four mouths had a breathing spell.

Up to this time the talk had been a staccato performance between mouthfuls:

"Yes—came near smashing a donkey—don't care if I do— no—no gravy" (Sculptor). "Let me put an extra bubble in your glass" (Knight). "These fish are as firm as the Adirondack trout" (Man from the Quarter). "More cream—thank you. Marie!" (Knight, of course) "more butter." "Donkey wasn't the only thing we missed—grazed a baby carriage and—" (Scribe).

"I'm going to try a red ibis after luncheon and a miller for a tail fly—pass the melon" (Man from the Quarter): That sort of hurried talk without logical beginning or ending.

But now each man had a comfortable chair, and filled it with shoulders hidden deep in its capacious depths, and legs straight out, only the arms and hands free enough to be within reach of the match-safe and thimble glasses. And with the ease and comfort of it all the talk itself slowed down to a pace more in harmony with that peace which passeth all understanding— unless you've a seat at the table.

The several masters of the outdoor school were now called up, their merits discussed and their failings hammered: Thaulow, Sorolla y Bastida, the new Spanish wonder, whose exhibition the month before had astonished and delighted Paris: the Glasgow school; Zorn, Sargent, Winslow Homer— all the men of the direct, forceful school, men who swing their brushes from their spines instead of their finger-tips—were slashed into and made mincemeat of or extolled to the skies. Then the "patty-pats," with their little dabs of yellow, blue, and red, in imitation of the master Monet; the "slick and slimies," and the "woollies"—the men who essayed the vague, mysterious, and obscure—were set up and knocked down one after the other, as is the custom with all groups of painters the world over when the never-ending question of technique is tossed into the middle of the arena.

Outdoor work next came into review and the discomforts and hardships a painter must go through to get what he is after, the Man from the Quarter defending the sit-by-the-fire fellows.

"No use making a submarine diver of yourself, Knight," he growled. "Go and look at it and then come home and paint the impression and put something of yourself into it."

Knight threw his head back and laughed. "I'd rather put the brook in—all of it."

"But I don't see why you've got to get soaked to the skin every time you want to make a sketch."

ICH

DER Nordostwind war an diesem Morgen sehr frisch und trieb die See lebhaft vor sich her; aber die „*Denver*" ging in ihrer Bulldoggenmanier auf jeden von ihnen los, vergrub ihre weiße Nase darin und überschüttete die Kämme derjenigen, die besonders ungestüm waren, mit glitzerndem Gischt über ihrem Vordeck. Im Osten begann die Oktobersonne gerade über die Meereslinie zu lugen, während im Norden die große Berginsel Madeira lag, die sich durch die magische Berührung des Lichts bereits von einem Phantomgrau in dieses lebendige Grün verwandelte, das so lieb ist in den Augen eines Seemanns. Bald zeigten sich Lebenszeichen; In jedem der Täler, die den Berghang zerfurchten, konnte man ein Dorf erkennen, während gelbe Villen die bewaldeten Hänge säumten. In einer Bucht am Südhang, weiß im Morgensonnenlicht, lag die Stadt Funchal, vor der wie ein riesiger Wächter knietief ein hoch aufragender Felsen mit einer Festung stand, der an eine Burg auf einem Felsen erinnerte Schachbrett.

Mr. Keegan, Oberbootsmannmaat der *Denver*, und sein Freund, Jimmy Legs, [1] der Waffenmeister, saßen auf der Wetterseite des Vorschiffs, unter dem vorderen Acht-Zoll-Turm, mit den Krägen ihrer Die Cabanjacken waren bis über die Ohren hochgekrempelt und rauchten morgens. Mr. Keegan hatte ein scharfes Gespür für das Schöne, und bei solchen Gelegenheiten pflegte er bis zu eine Stunde lang schweigend zu sitzen. Der Waffenmeister, der ein Mann auf dem Zwischendeck war, genoss es, zuzusehen, wie die Wellen über dem Bug brachen, obwohl ihn dieses Vergnügen nicht selten ein Wasser und eine Pfeife Tabak kostete.

[1] Der Name, der dem Waffenmeister an Bord eines Schiffes gegeben wurde.

Mr. Keegan war ein junger Mann mit rötlichem Haar und kleinen, ausdruckslosen blauen Augen, und sein Vorname war Dennis. Er hatte ein rundes, volles Gesicht, ungewöhnlicherweise auf einer Seite wegen des großen Stücks marineblauem Pfropfen, das es immer aufblähte. Ich habe gesagt, dass er Oberbootsmannsmaat der *Denver war*, weil er in der Abteilung so bekannt war und auch seinen Lohn als solchen bezog. Tatsächlich ließen sich der Status von Herrn Keegan und der Umfang seines Einflusses an Bord dieses Schiffes jedoch ebenso schwer definieren wie die in den neuen Vorschriften festgelegten Pflichten des Kapitäns. Sein Freund, der Waffenmeister, beriet ihn in allen wichtigen Angelegenheiten; die Unteroffiziere des Schiffes mischten sich nie in irgendetwas ein, was er tun

Doch zu seinem großen Unbehagen schien Miss Inglefield die Situation nicht im Geringsten zu begreifen.

"Wer bist du?" sie forderte mit einem Anflug von Ungeduld.

„Ich bin der Waffenmeister der *Denver*, Miss", antwortete er in einem Ton verletzter Würde.

„Aber was sind die Befehle, von denen Sie sprechen? Das verstehe ich nicht ganz."

Was waren die Befehle? Aus verschiedenen Dingen, die er in Miss Inglefields Unterhaltung und Verhalten bemerkt hatte, begann dem Waffenmeister der Verdacht zu dämmern, dass sie vorher keine Ahnung von der Mitteilung gehabt hatte, die er ihr mitteilen wollte. Dies war ein Punkt, den Herr Keegan nicht angesprochen hatte. Er steckte in einer Zwickmühle. Sich jetzt zurückzuziehen, könnte Mr. Penningtons Ehre verletzen und darüber hinaus die Dinge für ihn, den Waffenmeister, äußerst unangenehm machen. Aber wenn Mr. Keegan zufällig einen Fehler gemacht hätte, würde das Weitermachen Mr. Pennington in eine Schwierigkeit bringen, deren Schwere der Waffenmeister vorher nicht bedacht hatte. Aber sein Vertrauen in Mr. Keegan und die Angst vor seinem Unmut überwogen schließlich.

„Sehen Sie, Miss", begann er, „der Grund, warum ich hierher gekommen bin und nicht Dennis, war folgender: Ich kenne zufällig die Seenora, ebenso wie die Küche für Sie, und Dennis hat gesagt, ich solle das erzählen hier zur Seenora, und die Seenora —"

„Hat Mr. Pennington eine Nachricht geschickt?" Miss Inglefield unterbrach sich verzweifelt.

"Eine Notiz!" wiederholte der Waffenmeister abfällig; „Er hat mich oder Dennis noch nie mit einer Notiz beleidigt, Fräulein."

„Dann machen Sie bitte schnell weiter", sagte sie; „Ich kann jeden Moment angerufen werden."

„Es gibt nichts außer diesem, Miss", begann er, allerdings keineswegs, um sich zu beeilen: „Mr. Penningtons Zeit auf dem Schiff ist heute abgelaufen, und er hat Tickets für *zwei Personen gekauft*" – der Waffenmeister fand die Schlussfolgerung sehr erfreulich und betonte die Ziffer – „auf dem Dampfer, der heute Abend abfährt." Dann geht er zu Dennis Keegan, der in jungen Jahren auf vielen Kreuzfahrten mit ihm war, und auch an vielen schwierigen Orten, und er sagt: „Keegan, hier oben auf dem Hügel hinter Funchal lebt eine junge Dame …" „Was Sie heute Abend gerne mitnehmen würden, Mr. Pennington", wirft Dennis ein, „aber es gibt wieder bestimmte Gründe, dass Sie raufgehen und sie selbst holen." Mr. Pennington sah einigermaßen überrascht aus, aber, Herr! Miss, er sollte wissen, dass da nicht viel los ist, was Dennis nicht vorhat. „Nun, Sir", fuhr Dennis fort, ohne ihm Zeit zu geben, etwas zu sagen, „alles, was Sie tun müssen, ist, diese Angelegenheit hier mir und Chimmy zu überlassen" – das bin ich, Fräulein – „und wenn das so ist, junge Dame." Ich bin nicht bereit, mit Ihnen zu gehen, wann auch immer Sie sagen, es wird nicht unsere Schuld sein, Sir."'

Der Waffenmeister hielt inne und wischte sich mit seinem roten Taschentuch den Schweiß aus dem Gesicht, während er Miss Inglefield die ganze Zeit ängstlich beobachtete. Sie hatte während dieses Vortrags still daneben gesessen, aber er konnte an ihrem Atem, der schnell kam und ging, erkennen, dass sie jetzt aufgeregt war, und sein Vertrauen in Mr. Keegans Urteilsvermögen verdoppelte sich. Wenn die junge Dame in diesem Fall so sehr verliebt war, wie diese Symptome den Anschein erweckten, war der von ihm eingeschlagene Weg offensichtlich höchst gerechtfertigt. Der Waffenmeister war immer davon ausgegangen, dass eine kleine Ausflüchte für einen guten Zweck nicht schädlich sei. Offensichtlich gab es in Miss Inglefield einen ziemlichen mentalen Kampf. Ein- oder zweimal schien sie kurz davor, etwas zu sagen, und dann ihre Meinung zu ändern. Zu diesem Zeitpunkt hörte man eine herzliche männliche Stimme, die laut aus dem Garten oben rief:

„Eleanor!"

Miss Inglefield stand auf.

„Komm, Papa", antwortete sie; aber zum Erstaunen des Waffenmeisters zeigte sie nicht die geringste Beunruhigung. Sie ging langsam auf die Stufe zu, den Kopf nachdenklich gesenkt; dann richtete sie sich plötzlich zu ihrer vollen Größe auf und blickte ihn an.

„Um wie viel Uhr wird Mr. Pennington hier sein?" sie verlangte.

„Um halb zwölf, am Hintertor, Fräulein", antwortete er und bezweifelte, dass er richtig gehört hatte.

„Sag ihm, dass ich bereit sein werde", sagte sie; und bevor er antworten konnte, war sie zwischen den Weinreben verschwunden.

Der Waffenmeister stand einen Moment da und schaute ihr nach, dann verließ er den Garten und hielt wachsam Ausschau nach Mr. Inglefield. Nach einiger Mühe fand er seine Bulla-Carta vor einem verirrten Weinladen, der in die Mauer eingebaut war und in den er sich auf der Suche nach seinem Jehus stürzte. Es ist zu bezweifeln, ob einer von ihnen die erlesenen maritimen Beschimpfungen verstand, mit denen er sie unparteiisch überhäufte, weil sie sich versteckten; aber sie bedeuteten ihm mit beruhigender Großzügigkeit, in das Fahrzeug zu steigen, und machten sich

„Sei kein Narr, Jack", sagte er. „Siehst du nicht, dass du jetzt alles hast, was du tun kannst, um um halb elf dort oben zu sein? Das Mädchen hat doppelt so viel Sand wie du."

„Wenn Sie jetzt nicht anfangen, Sir", warf Mr. Keegan ein, „hat es überhaupt keinen Sinn, zu gehen."

„Keegan", sagte Pennington – und die Kühle seiner Rede und die Beherrschung seiner Stimme beeindruckten beide, als er sprach – „Ich kenne dich jetzt seit fast neun Jahren und du bist einer der besten Freunde, die ich habe." hatte jemals. Als ich jünger war, hast du mich aus zwei oder drei schwierigen Situationen herausgeholt, was ich wahrscheinlich nicht vergessen werde. In diesen neun Jahren hast du mich nie getäuscht, und ich glaube nicht, dass du dazu in der Lage bist; aber nach allem, was ich über Miss Inglefield weiß, halte ich es für mehr als wahrscheinlich, dass der Waffenmeister sie missverstanden hat. Trotzdem möchte ich Ihnen dafür danken." Dann wandte er sich an Morgan und fuhr fort: „Siehst du nicht, Holländer, wie unmöglich es wäre, das zu tun, was Keegan heute Abend vorschlägt, selbst wenn es keinen Fehler gibt?" Natürlich werde ich jetzt auf den nächsten Dampfer warten. Aber es gibt bestimmte Dinge, an die man denken muss – alle auf ihre Art sehr notwendig und in zweieinhalb Stunden nur sehr schwer zu bewerkstelligen."

"Herr. „Pennington", sagte Mr. Keegan ernst, „wenn Chimmy hier einen Fehler gemacht hat, dann bin ich bereit, mich morgen zum Marine Corps zu melden." Das war nachdrücklicher als jeder Eid, den sich Mr. Keegan vorstellen konnte. Dann schloss er mit einer Endgültigkeit, die weitere Bedenken zunichte machte: „Mit einem Himmelspiloten wird es keinen Ärger geben; Auf dem Schiff, mit dem Sie unterwegs sind, ist einer, der sagt, er werde alles in Ordnung bringen und bis dahin schweigen. Und was die Einzelheiten angeht, Sie können nichts erwähnen, was nicht behoben ist, Sir."

Daraufhin nahm Morgan den Reisekoffer und ging hinaus, gefolgt von Mr. Keegan und Pennington, letzterer in einem schwer zu beschreibenden Geisteszustand, der weder für Morgan noch für Mr. Keegan verständlich war. Mr. Keegan hatte drei Pferde herangezogen, eines davon bestieg er selbst, während Morgan ein anderes bestieg, und Pennington stieg mechanisch auf das dritte. Sie starteten so schnell, wie es das Gesetz erlaubte, und die Läufer folgten schweigend an ihrer Seite. Das Burroughs's Hotel lag auf einer Anhöhe im Westen der Stadt, während die Inglefield-Villa an den Hängen im Norden lag. Die Straße führte ein Stück an den hohen Klippen entlang, die den Hafen säumen, wo die Ankerlichter der Schiffe funkelten und tanzten. Pennington konnte die *Denver* an ihren weißen Seiten und ihrer kompromisslosen, massigen Form erkennen, die durch die elektrischen

Lichter des großen schwarzen Dampfers, der kaum einen Steinwurf von ihr entfernt war, sichtbar wurde. Aber seine Gedanken galten nicht der *Denver*; er blickte auf den Rauch, der bereits aus den Rohren des Dampfers strömte; es war Zeit – kaum zwei Stunden. Und vielleicht dann: „Was für ein Unsinn!" rief er halb laut vor sich hin. Es konnte nicht möglich sein, dass dieses Mädchen, das ihn noch vor fünf Monaten so entschieden abgelehnt hatte, einem solch verrückten Unterfangen wie diesem überhaupt zustimmen würde, geschweige denn, es vorzuschlagen. Dennoch schien Mr. Keegan wie immer selbstsicher zu sein und zu wissen, was er tat. Dieser würdige Mann stand an der Spitze der Kolumne und pfiff leise eine ziemlich zweifelhafte Stimme, die er im Jahr zuvor in einem Bowery-Theater aufgeschnappt hatte. Mr. Keegans Reitkunst war nicht die beste; Als das Tempo jedoch zu einem Trab beschleunigte, gelang es ihm, weiterzumachen, und er tröstete sich mit dem Gedanken, dass es zu dunkel war, als dass die Dago-Heeler Kritik hätten üben können. Als sie die Stadt erreichten, waren die engen Gassen fast menschenleer und die Weinhandlungen begannen zu schließen. Mr. Keegan zügelte sein Pferd und wartete darauf, dass die anderen herankamen.

„Dieser Ticketverkäufer muss festgehalten werden, Mr. Morgan", sagte er.

Morgan war klug genug, die Bedeutung dieser Tatsache zu erkennen und auch zu erkennen, dass sie bessere Erfolgsaussichten hatten, wenn Mr. Keegan mit Pennington nach oben ging. Obwohl es für ihn eine bittere Enttäuschung war, sich an dem Versuch nicht wesentlicher beteiligt zu haben, als den Agenten „festzuhalten", gab er sofort nach und war davongeritten, bevor Pennington Einwände erheben konnte.

„Nun, Sir", bemerkte Mr. Keegan, „wir haben keine Zeit, diesen Hügel hinaufzufahren."

Sie polterten unter Missachtung eines Stadtgesetzes über die Steine und machten sich bald auf den Weg. Abgesehen von einer gelegentlichen Lampe am Eingang einer Villa war es so dunkel, dass sie die hohen Mauern auf beiden Seiten kaum erkennen konnten. Ein- oder zweimal hätte Pennington fast beschlossen, umzukehren, aber Mr. Keegan drängte so eifrig voran, als könne es keinen Zweifel am Ausgang geben, dass Pennington ihm weiter folgte. Als sie unter einem der schwachen Lichter in der Wand vorbeifuhren, schoss ein Schlitten vorbei, in dem Pennington, mit großer Selbstzufriedenheit rauchend, zwei Mitglieder der Freiheitspartei *von Denver erkennen konnte.*

„Das hast du gut hinbekommen, Keegan", sagte Pennington, als er neben ihm anhielt.

„Chimmy macht das, Sir", antwortete Mr. Keegan bescheiden; „Er ist da oben und fängt an." Und dann fügte er mit einem Anflug von Befriedigung

Nun geschah es, dass der Waffenmeister, der sich etwas weiter unten am Hügel verborgen gehalten hatte, den Tumult hörte und von der Vorstellung besessen wurde, dass sein Freund Mr. Keegan in Schwierigkeiten geriet. Er kam genau in diesem Moment am Tatort an.

„Nun, Mr. Inglefield", fuhr Mr. Keegan fort und warf einen Blick auf die Gesichter an der Laterne, „das hier ist kein Ort, um über private Angelegenheiten zu sprechen; Aber wenn Sie sich die Mühe machen, mit uns einzutreten, werden ich und Chimmy versuchen, Ihnen hier einen kurzen Bericht darüber zu geben, Sir."

„Kommen Sie auf jeden Fall herein, wenn Sie etwas Licht in diese schurkische Angelegenheit bringen können", sagte Mr. Inglefield, nahm die Laterne und ging voran zum Haus. Die anderen folgten.

„Dennis", sagte der Waffenmeister zu Mr. Keegan und zog ihn am Ärmel, „es hat keinen Sinn, dass ich da reingehe; Du weißt, wie man mit dem Alten umgeht. Ich werde die Seera für den kleinen Anruf bezahlen, den ich heute Nachmittag verpasst habe."

Mr. und Mrs. Pennington, bzw. der Waffenmeister, wussten nie genau, wie Mr. Keegan während der halben Stunde, die er mit ihm zusammen war, „mit dem Alten umgegangen" war. Mr. Keegan würde es natürlich nie verraten. Als er vom Waffenmeister zu diesem Thema befragt wurde, konnte er nur dazu gebracht werden, Folgendes zu sagen:

„Er ging hinein wie ein Löwe und kam wieder heraus wie ein Lamm, nicht wahr, Chimmy?"

Der Waffenmeister gab dies zu.

„Nun, Chimmy", antwortete er und blinzelte feierlich mit seinen kleinen Augen, „das ist alles dran."

In der Dienstzeitschrift, die in New York erscheint, erschien folgender Artikel:

„Eine äußerst interessante und neuartige Hochzeit fand am Donnerstag, dem 31. Oktober, in Funchal, Madeira, an Bord des Dampfers *Southampton* der Union Line statt. Fähnrich John R. Pennington, USN, heiratete Miss Eleanor Inglefield, Tochter von Robert Inglefield, Esq., aus Ravenside, der lange und hervorragend mit dem britischen diplomatischen Dienst verbunden war. Das Brautpaar reiste sofort nach England. Aufgrund der überstürzten Abreise von Mr. Pennington kam die Hochzeit selbst für seine Offiziersbrüder von *Denver eine Überraschung dar* . Das junge Paar ist jetzt in Newport, wo Fähnrich Pennington stationiert ist; und es versteht sich, dass der Vater der Braut den Winter bei ihnen verbringen wird."

Der Bericht stimmte, denn bevor die Denver Funchal verließ, war die Inglefield-Villa geschlossen, und die Senhora regierte dort als Oberhaupt; und Herr Inglefield war nach Newport gegangen, um seinen neuen Schwiegersohn zu besuchen und seinen ersten Besuch in den Vereinigten Staaten abzustatten.

Mr. Keegan besitzt jetzt eine große Goldkette, die an einer großen Golduhr befestigt ist, auf die er sehr stolz ist und die er bei allen Gelegenheiten trägt. Auf der Außenseite des Gehäuses befindet sich das sehr schön eingravierte Monogramm „DK" und auf der Innenseite eine geheimnisvolle Inschrift, deren Bedeutung Herr Keegan nie preisgegeben hat, die aber vermutlich Ausdruck der ewigen Dankbarkeit zweier Menschen ist .

Auch sein Freund, der Waffenmeister, wurde nicht vergessen.

MR. WINSTON CHURCHILL hat, wie Mr. WISTER und Mr. CRAWFORD , einen tieferen Anspruch auf den Namen „amerikanischer Autor", als Wohnort und Themenwahl vermuten lassen, da das Blut Neuenglands auf beiden Seiten bis ins 16. Jahrhundert zurückreicht, im Süden Geburt und eine Ausbildung an der United States Naval Academy in Annapolis waren in seiner Ausrüstung vereint. Doch nach nur kurzer Dienstzeit bei der Marine legte er sein Amt nieder und folgte endgültig seinem literarischen Geschmack. Er war für kurze Zeit beim *Army and Navy Journal* , während dieser Zeit erschien seine erste Kurzgeschichte „Mr. Keegan's Elopement" wurde im *Century Magazine veröffentlicht* . Herr CHURCHILL wurde Redakteur des *Cosmopolitan Magazine* , verließ dies jedoch wieder, um mehr Zeit für kontinuierliche Originalarbeit zu haben als für die Routineaufgaben, die mit einer monatlichen Zeitschriftenerlaubnis verbunden sind.

Sein erstes Buch erschien 1897: „The Celebrity", geschrieben im Stil der lebhaftesten Komödie; Aber selbst dann war der erste Teil seiner Romanreihe gut, der charakteristische Phasen der gesellschaftlichen Entwicklung Amerikas abdeckt und nach Fertigstellung ein Bild des nationalen Lebens liefern wird, das nicht nur seinesgleichen sucht, sondern in seiner Breite und Gesamtheit noch nie versucht wurde im Gange.

Sicherlich „Die Berühmtheit", obwohl anerkannt als –

Prelude

Many times I have been called a story teller, and throughout my life I have often been accused of being a "Nut-Magnate". I seem to find myself in what some people might call strange and unusual circumstances. I have often asked the Lord, "If I have to go through this situation, would you please let me learn something from it?" And I have learned from them. Through my teaching and ministering of God's word the BIBLE. I often use some of these experiences as examples in order to try to get my points across and try to help others better understand our relationships between each other as well as our relationship to God. Quiet often people have ask me, "Why don't you write a book of those stories? After giving it much thought; this is the first collection of some of those stories and poems I have written. Please join me as I ponder the question, "What was I Thinking?"

ourselves just like Dudley Badd. We are in a position that we didn't even realize that we were in. Covered with the filth of the world, rolling in sins. Weak disorientated, thinking we can't let go. We lay there trapped calling for help but not helping ourselves.

The first time Dudley took a drink he never imagined that one morning he would wake up underneath a cabin floor in the woods holding a chicken by the leg. If he had thought would happen you could believe that he never would have taken another drink. Would you? Of course not, but the drink is not the only thing that can distance you from the Lord. Today, look at your life. Where are you? What is the thing that you are clinging to instead of Christ? Your hands and heart are not big enough to grasp more than one thing at a time. Which will it be? Where are things that you are clinging too taken you? Are you holding them? Or are they holding you?

It's often not the messenger that we reject. It is the message. As annoying as an alarm usually is, we have them to alert us to danger. Taking heed to an alarm in time will save your life.

1Thes 4:16 "For the Lord himself shall descend from heaven with a shout, with the voice of the archangel, and with the trump of God: and the dead in Christ shall rise first: Then we which are alive and remain shall be caught up together with them in the clouds, to meet the Lord in the air: and so shall we ever be with the Lord. Wherefore comfort one another with these words." There will be another call in the morning, the next time it will be the trump of the Lord, will it be a call that you will be excited about or just another rooster crowing in the night?

Chapter Three

FEED MY SHEEP

"Give me that hot dog," he screamed as he pushed me aside and tried to jerk the food from my hand. "Feed me, feed me," he cried.

I was sitting in front of Radio City Music Hall on the wall of the fountain in midtown Manhattan one day on my lunch break, when I decided to buy a hot dog from a nearby vendor. As usual, the sidewalks were crowded as the mass of people hurried along their way. As I waited my turn in line, I could not help but notice a well-groomed man of average dress looking to be in his mid-thirties. The man was leaning against a nearby wall and appeared to be waiting for someone. As I paid for my meal, he turned, straightened himself and started walking my way. When I took the hot dog and began to step away, the man suddenly sprang forward and grabbed my food. Immediately we began to tussle. As he tried to wrench the food from my hand, he began to scream "feed me, feed me" over and over again. I finally gained control of the situation and pulling away said without thinking, "Get your own food."

Behind me I heard the vendor say, "Leave my customer alone, I'll feed you." "No," he cried, "I want him to feed me." Quickly looking back to see why it had to be me, I found the man had disappeared into the crowd.

Suddenly I felt sick at heart. I had never been more disappointed in myself. In my pockets was more than enough money to feed twenty people hot dogs and all he wanted was just one. Acting on a natural human instinct, I hadn't wanted anyone taking something was mine. As I walked away, I immediately remembered the scripture in Hebrews 13:2 "Be not forgetful to entertain strangers: for thereby some have entertained angels unawares."

As I returned to my seat at the fountain wall my friend asked, "What was that all about?" "I don't know," I replied, "I'm really not sure." I have relived that scene over and over in my mind many times and still it haunts me.

been passed along for generations within her family and now and until she would pass them on they were hers. The only source of her joy, she would take them out often to look at the deteriorating patterns and view her image in their reflections. Not being able to afford a nice china hutch Emma kept them in the bottom two drawers of her infant son's chest of drawers.

Sometime past midnight on the night in question Emma awakened to the sound of her baby crying. Opening the top drawer of his chest to get some dry clothing, Emma froze. There was Herman, sound asleep, curled in the baby's pajamas. Slowly she closed the drawer. Rushing to her bedroom she began to shake Arlo awake screaming, he is in the baby's room, he is in the baby's room. Coming wide-awake and thinking an intruder was in the house Arlo grabbed his pistol from the nightstand and rushed into the bedroom. Quickly surveying the room, seeing no intruder he asked with a puzzled look on his face. " Who, where, where did he go?"

"He is in that drawer" Emma screamed. Slowly opening the drawer Arlo saw Herman. Hearing all the noise Herman opened his right eye for a look, recognizing that it was only Arlo. Herman closed his eyes and went right back to sleep. Gently Arlo placed the muzzle of the pistol against Herman's head and pulled the trigger.

Now asleep in the next room Arlo could not hear the cries of despair as Ema went through each drawer in the chest trying to find at least one piece of her beloved china that wasn't shattered.

In Matthew the thirteenth chapter Jesus cautions us about destroying the wheat by trying to pull the tares out of the field. He wanted us to know that there are going to be some rats in the church. And that there will always be some moving in and moving out. I'm talking about the two-legged kind. It is not our job to try to rid the church of them for in doing so we stand the risk of destroying far more than the things that they will harm. After all the church is not ours it is His. The church is more precious to Him than Emma's fine china was to her. And if we destroy it like Arlo did the china we will not feel the same loss that Jesus would. After all he went to Calvary for each of us. It is not his will that any should perish. Our place is to keep the church open and alive and let the master do the sorting out in his own good time. The hour is growing late and as the midnight hour approaches is not the time to go on Safari.

pain, exhausted hurting and broken, words alone mean absolutely nothing. For a long time now, my wife and I have tried to live our life in such a fashion as to help others without any thought of recompense or reward. But I have been guilty myself of just offering words instead of actions. I have prided myself in being compassionate and reaching out to others with my kind words. Words are easy. Words are free. Words cost you nothing and words alone are so empty. When you are surrounded by darkness and you don't know where the next attack is coming from, words can be as big an enemy as anything else. If Nicholas had kept his mouth shut that night, he would have lived another Christmas. But the reaction was to the sound of his words, not to his message. If the light had been turned on, his words would have been accepted as friendly and comforting; not scared and threatening. Let us first let the light of Jesus show in our actions, before we ever put the words into the situation. If we let our light so shine before men they will glorify the Father and He will draw all men to him.

Chapter Eight

THE HANG OF THINGS

The pain in my side began to rouse me awake, it was hard to believe that I could hurt in so many places at once. There it was again a sharp piercing pain. in my side.....Wait, I hear voices .... where am I.... who is here?

" Well, are you alive or not?" Mark ask as he gently nudged me in the ribs once more. With sudden realization it all came back to me. Moments earlier, hanging from the holly tree limb high above I knew I had come to the end. The only way to save myself was to let go of something very precious to me. And I just didn't want to do that. Now laying here in all this pain, I wished that I had dropped the load earlier.

The much anticipated arrival of my good friend found me sick in the bed with the influenza. The day of the hunting we had planned over six months ago had finally

arrived and he had traveled across two states to join me. Pride keeping me from good sense, I was entirely to macho to listen to reason. Besides I had spent a small fortune on new camouflage clothes, hunting license and other misc. equipment. And on top of that, I had a brand new gun to try out too. No way I was going to stay home.

As we began to walk through dark woods, I realized I had made a mistake. Leaving my friend in his deer stand, I traveled only a few hundred yards before I grew weary. There in the trail in front of me was a huge holly tree so I decided that this was far enough and I climbed it. Settling down in the top of the tree, I was quite comfortable until I passed out. As the world disappeared beneath, me I wildly lashed out and miraculously caught hold of a limb with my left hand.. The trouble was, I to far from the trunk to reach it with my feet. There were no other limbs close by and I was holding my new gun with my right hand.

For some time I managed to hold on, not knowing what to do, I just didn't want to drop the gun. Finally the will to survive took over, only then it was to late. As my strength began to fade, I threw the rifle at a nearby bush in hopes it would survive, and reached for and thus insuring our safety. As I rolled over to go to sleep I thought of the fear I had as a young boy. *"Fear of the Timber wolves"*.

Sometime later, around three A.M. I awoke and could see one young man still sitting by the fire with a large stick in his hand. Thinking he might want some company I left my tent and walked to the fire. To my surprise he was sound asleep sitting upright in the chair. Before I had a chance to consider my actions… sometime I just can't help myself. I dropped to my knees and crawled alongside of the night guard. Emitting a loud growling sound I attacked his leg in my best wild dog imitation.

The bloodcurdling scream that filled the night woke every camper on that end of the lake. And may have alerted the air raid personal at the nearest town several miles away. It wasn't just that it was loud, but it started so high in the air and continued as my young friend plummeted back to earth swinging wildly with his arms in every direction. At least he didn't land in the fire.

Fear is like that, we often react before we actually come under attack. Someone wiser than myself figured it out years ago when he said, " We have nothing to fear but fear itself." I personally can take a small thing and begin to toy with it in my mind until it begins to grow. Kneading it softly over and over it begins to grow. I add the yeast of the unknown future, the flour of past failures and the milk of insecurity. And before long the bread of fear begins to rise until it begins to spill over the side of the container and begins to get on to everything that I am involved with. I don't believe that God is pleased with us living a life full of fear. He has asked us to put our trust in him.

The barnyard was dark when the leader of the Wolf Pak came silently back to the scene of the crime. As he approached a rabbit hutch, suddenly jaws of a steel trap gripped his front right foot. Jumping backwards his back left foot was caught in another trap. Spinning wildly his front left foot was caught next and then stepping to the side his back right foot became ensnared also. Watching in disbelief as his friends abandoned him Wolfe sat down on his haunches in defeat. All his plans came to an abrupt end as the last trap closed on his backside.

This was exactly where we found him the next morning when we out the barnyard to check on things. The brown black and gray dog seemed so small cowering there dirty and afraid. It sure is funny how things can change overnight. Suddenly the fear that I had known for so long was gone. No longer afraid I only felt sorry for the animal. His bark had certainly been bigger than his bite.

Revelation 20:1-3 "And I saw an angel come down from heaven, having the key of the bottomless pit and a great chain in his hand. And he laid hold on the dragon, that old serpent, which is the Devil, and Satan, and bound him a thousand years. And cast him into the bottomless pit, and shut him up, and set a seal upon him, that he should deceive the nations no more..."

I am tired of our people, children of the Most High God living in fear. The word of God tells us that it will only take one angel with one chain to bind the enemy and cast him into the pit. The Roaring Dragon will be gone and our fears with him. If you are someone that has been listening to his howling in the darkness it is time to quit. When the light of Jesus Christ shines on the fears you hold on to things come back into perspective. Big problems become small. Sicknesses give way to healing. Trials turn into victories.

"The Lord is my light and my salvation; whom shall I fear? The Lord is the strength of my life; of whom shall I be afraid? When the wicked, even mine enemies and my foes, came upon me to eat up my flesh, they stumbled and fell. Though an host should encamp against me, my heart shall not fear: though war should rise against me, in this will I be confident. One thing have I desired of the Lord, that will I seek after; that I may dwell in the house of the Lord all the days of my life, to behold the beauty of the Lord, and to enquire in his temple". Psalms 28:1-4

If we are determined that we are going to hide in the house under the covers? Then why don't we hide in the Lord's house under the cover of his protecting hand? And see the beautiful things that he can do with the things we fear. Remember old Wolfe's bark is a lot bigger than his bite.

Last year my nephew kept me from stepping on a velvet tailed rattle snake that was so well concealed that my next step would have landed right on top of him. When I asked him how he was able to see it when I didn't. He told me he had seen the snake blink his eyes and it was only that movement that alerted him.

As I was driving home from the woods last weekend I began to reminisce of the above mentioned situations. A few hours earlier while still in the forest a friend of mine and myself had an invigorating square dance with a copper head moccasin.

I arrived at the camp and had visited with the others a while and then began preparation to transport a tripod deer stand to the area I had planned to hunt. Before I left I asked, "Have any of you guys seen any snakes out here?" Everyone assured me that none had been seen by anyone. With that peace of mind I left the camp. Driving an old three-wheeler with no breaks I descended the long hill from camp, the weight of the deer stand pushed me down the hill faster than I intended to go. Ahead of me crossing the trail was a six-foot long blue runner (snake). As I was trying to stop to keep from hitting the snake I envisioned the large knobby front tire slinging the snake up onto the bike and into my lap. In spite of the briars and thorns in the area there are now two parallel trails along that section of the path. I could not stop the bike. As the others joined me again they assured me that they had not seen that snake either and wondered why I felt it necessary to have two trails through the briar patch instead of only one.

After all the joking and kidding we loaded the deer stand on our shoulders and began carrying it through the woods. My friend had the front and I had the rear. The way we had to weave our arms through the braces and shoulder the load did not allow a quick process to loose ourselves from its burden and lay it back down. After a short walk I looked down and noticed that my friend had just stepped over a snake in the path and now one more step would put me on top of it.

Immediately I cried out, "don't move there is a snake!" At the same time I instinctively began to back away from the offending reptile. Now as I backed away shouting over and over, "don't move, don't move." I began pulling my friend back into harm's way. Realizing He was now going back towards the snake he began moving forward to escape, thus moving me once again towards the snake. This process was repeated over and over again. The whole time I was screaming out, "don't move" and yet pulling him backwards. Finally the snake had enough and ran away leaving us to dance alone.

It was then that I realized my actions were not consistent with my words. Driving home I wondered if we as Christians don't often do the same thing. We tell others about the love of God and how he is concerned with our everyday wellbeing and how through Him we are over comers. And yet we by our actions clearly tell them that we don't believe it ourselves. We tell them Jesus can deliver them from their sins and yet with our actions we pull them back into a life style of unbelief. Thus saying it is ok to do the things that I like to do but the things that you enjoy are wrong. Instead of lining ourselves up with what the word of God says we pick and choose the things that we are willing to lay aside and thus say one thing and let our actions send a different message.

It is possible that we can dance around the snake long enough that we began to lose our fear of it. Before long we will want to pick it up, maybe have a drink with it. And then one day without realizing it we will be in love with it.

In 1972 during the Madi-Gra festival in New Orleans I stumbled into a witchcraft shop just off of the French Quarter. Thinking it was a novelty shop my friend and I curiously entered. Hearing chanting and music we were drawn to the back of the store. In the back room there were a number of people kneeling on the floor worshiping Satan, and for the first time in my life I realized that he really did have a people who worshipped him. Gripped with fear I turned to leave, it was then that I mistakenly entered the room that contained the lady with the snake.

I don't believe that one morning you just happen to wake up and say, "Today I am going to make love to a snake". It is a process that takes place over a period of time. A process produced by our actions. Day by day letting ourselves become conditioned to the presence of the offender. And then before we know it we are no longer afraid. Instead of being frightened by just the blink of the snake's eye we are able to hold and caress it.

instructions for us. Why don't we get into God's word and read it for ourselves. Then we will know what he wants us to do. And how he wants us to react to the situations we find ourselves in. I really believe the Lord wants us to seek his face about issues in our lives rather than to just follow prescribed methods.

Your walk with God is unique to you. No one else has the relationship that you do. It is a beautiful and wonderful thing. Enjoy it pursue it. Don't turn this awesome experience into one like the "Tribal Dance of the Hairy Neck Mud Stomper" I described above. The method for removing hair down the back of your neck is certainly different from the procedure to remove mud from your boots. And so it is with every situation life throws your way. Don't try to pattern the actions of a mediocre Christian to obtain the walk that God has called you to take. Ask God what he would have you to do, and then do it. Then watch and see how wonderfully He will work the situations out.

Chapter Eighteen

SCARED TO DEATH

The moment he paused, his troubles began to multiply. Shrouded in the mist of an early morning fog, decisions were hard to make. In the dim light it was impossible to tell which would be wiser to venture forward or to turn around and go back. If evil had a smell, possibly he smelled it. If evil made a sound, maybe he heard it. If evil had a body, he may have seen it. All I know is that he knew it was there, lurking somewhere in the shadows ready to attack at any moment. And that worried him.

As I watched from my vantage point high above, he stopped on his journey. Quickly looking from right to left and back again he began to tremble. Slowly he sat down right in the well-traveled path. As his trembling increased I puzzled over the situation. There he sat apparently normal and healthy, yet he shook. His whole body shook so violently he could no longer stand his limbs and head took on the appearance of a small bush in a turbulent windstorm. For a moment I thought it was my vision beginning to blur, only then did the shaking stop as he fell limp and seemingly lifeless to the ground. It was then that the beast mounted his attack. Without a fight, with no sign of a struggle his captor lifted him and with a couple of steps disappeared into the brush and was gone. Death is so final. Had he only continued closer to where I was, his attacker would have turned away.

1 Peter 5:8 says "Be sober, be vigilant for your adversary the devil, as a roaring lion walketh about seeking whom he may devour." This scripture did not say he *was* a roaring lion, but that that he *walks about* as a roaring lion. A lion's roar can strike fear in even the bravest of men. Fear is one of the devil's favorite tools to use. With this weapon in his arsenal, he only has to initiate the idea and we do the rest. Our imagination can take even the smallest of problems and with just a little attention nurture them into mighty beast of terror.

" I can't pay the bills."

"I can't be healed from this infirmity."

"My children are lost and will never find God.."

"I've failed God and could never be forgiven."

With powerful strokes of his wings the majestic eagle climbed higher and higher into the morning sky. The heat of the sun growing warmer and warmer the higher he climbed. Perched on his back, the young eagle dug his small talons into his father's back to hold on secure and comfortable. Then without warning it happened.

Suddenly the male eagle turned straight up in his flight purposely dropping the young eagle off of his back. Flapping his wings furiously the young eagle fought the empty space around him. Not knowing how to fly he tumbled helplessly out of the sky.

Standing with their backs to the Red Sea the Israelites were scared and confused. Having been taken into slavery, like it or not they had settled into a consistent lifestyle. Then along comes a man called Moses, a stranger from the backside of the desert telling them that God had sent him to lead them out of captivity. Many people do not handle change easily. And the people of God are no exception. Pharaoh's army rapidly closing the gap behind them and the Red Sea in front of them, people began to whine and complain. Then only to make matters worse a storm came rushing across the mountains. Dark clouds rolled in and the wind began to blow. Dust and debris started to fill the air as the desert sand stung their faces. As the hurricane force wind moved across the crowds of people and into the sea, both animals and people crowded together heads down and discouraged the mass of people huddled. As one unit, they began to slowly move forward not really conscious that they were going somewhere.

Only those people closest to the man of God saw him as he lifted his hands over the sea. Surely some of the people nearest to the Prophet noticed as the waters parted and the wind blew the dry sand into a pathway in front of the multitude. Although many did not see it, the people moved forward, one small step at a time. Heads down, eyes filled with sand, heartbroken they moved. Thinking that they were just drawing closer to seek protection from the storm many of them failed to notice the walls of water moving away before them.

Later as the wind died and the people cleared their eyes they were amazed to find themselves across the Sea from where they had started when the storm began.

As in most miracles, those who participate often do not realize that it is happening until it is over. While the problem is apparent they often feel forsaken and abandoned by God. It is only much later that they realize "that all things" do "work together for them that love the Lord".

This past year I experienced change in a big way. Within a couple of weeks' time period everything that I depended on for stability vanished around me. The position I had as a senior manager at a large Engineering Firm was eliminated during a corporate downsizing program. And the first new job that I could find was a hundred miles from where we were located. The house that we were leasing was sold out from under us and we had to move quickly. And to top it all off, God called my good friend and pastor to a new field of work in another city.

Normally I could have handled all of this simply by just moving with the job. And seeing what happened next, except I knew that the Lord had called us to work in the place where we were. Pray as we might we could not feel the release from the place that we were called to labor.

So for a while we cried, prayed and drove back and forth one hundred miles each way every day to work. Felt dejected, forgotten, forsaken and confused. But we kept on working; often it felt like we were just going through the motions. You see we still loved Jesus, it's just that we couldn't understand why things were happening like they were.

As suddenly as things happened the first time things changed again. The phone call came from an unexpected direction. The dream job of a lifetime, ten minutes from home with better benefits and pay. More time off and surrounded by people I already knew. The very day that I took the new job the new pastor that our church elected came to town. A powerful man of God who quickly became a friend. In the same fashion that the sun burns the fog away as a new day begins, the confusion and disenchantment began to leave. I found myself stronger for having weathered another storm.

Whether it is an eagle teaching it's young to fly or God teaching a nation to trust in him. Change is often hard for everyone. God has a purpose for our every situation.

victim back to shore or calming a panicked person does not require heroic measures, but both save lives. Despite what most people believe rescues involve little more than lending a helping hand. Divers are taught never bring someone up too fast, do it in stages. The very air that kept them alive below, is the same air that will kill them on top. The expanding air in their bloodstream causes bubbles to collect in major arteries, which can cause the bends or a stroke. When a person is brought up slowly, it gives their body a chance to throw off excess nitrogen, so they can once again breathe and function on the surface. It should be the same way for Christians. Don't try to bring new Christians up to your level of standards and commitments too soon. Give them a chance to do some adjusting to their new environment. Let them learn to function at each new level as their experience with God grows.

Don't do anything fast! Mistakes are the results of not clearly thinking through your actions. We are told anything while diving that goes wrong can be fixed on the bottom, as well as at the surface. There is no reason to wait until a person is back on top and safe to correct the problems they are having. God too, will restore troubled lives, no matter what circumstance or problem you find yourself in. He will forgive and comfort your troubled heart even when you find yourself looking up just to see the bottom.

Rescue workers are taught *never to approach a person in distress from the rear.* Always let the person see you first, to get use to the idea that help has arrived. This causes the approach to have a calming effect and not call attention to how precarious the situation actually is. Panic is a serious liability. When the victim is located, always reach out and touch them. There is reassurance in the human touch.

Always use clear signals. Often we cause others to seek safety in places other than the Church, simply because we don't let them know

we are trying to help them instead of condemn them. When sharing air, diver's are told to never give their air away. Always hold the regulator and let the victim hold your hand. If they take your air supply, you might not get it back and both of you will drown. While we frequently try to meet people on their level to win them to Christ, we must never compromise our beliefs or let down our convictions.

Never let the person that you are helping rob you of your own spiritual strength, least you too should become lost. Once contact is made, never leave the victim to struggle alone. If more help is needed, **never go until the victim is calm and rational.** Just letting someone know that you are there for them may be enough. If you go for help to soon, they might not be where you left them when you return and by the time you find them again, it may be too late! As soon as contact is made have the person stop all their underwater activity and focus on gaining control of their breathing. This helps insure they get adequate air. In Psalms 46:10 it says, "Be still and know that I am God." We are often too busy trying to solve our own problems to listen to what God is trying to tell us. Loss of control will leave a person with the feeling of helplessness. This can build a wall between reality and rational thinking.

If complete control of the situation does not belong to the rescuer, then he should back away until calm is resumed. Self-preservation has to be number one. You cannot help someone when you're in trouble yourself. Often in haste to do good, we get to close to a given situation or too involved. Before we can be of help, we find ourselves struggling to save our own spiritual lives. When if done properly we could be helping to save someone else.

Listen to yourself, common sense will tell you you're in trouble, long before others notice.

When securing someone on the surface, the first action rescuers are taught should be to unlatch and discard or "ditch" the weights that the diver was using to keep him on the bottom. In Hebrews 12, we read to lay aside the weights and sins that so easily beset us. We too should discard known habits and items, that could hold us back from being all we can for Christ. Next, we should inflate a buoyancy device to help keep the person afloat until he has the strength to help himself. Still true today, as in that old gospel favorite "Love lifted me..." as Christians, love is still the best buoyancy device that we have to help keep new Christians afloat. We should use it as often as possible.

Most people don't realize that C.P.R. can be applied in the middle of the lake, as well as on the shore when you are trained. There is no need to drag around a dead person, resuscitate them and then help them to safety. It's much easier than trying to carry them and keep royal priesthood, an Holy nation then we should be functional in each of these rolls. A people who are different because of a love for God drives them to become obsessed with trying to do his will. A people who burn with the desire to win others to him with no thought of personal gain. A people who throughout their lives live in such a fashion as to allow Christ to permeate their every activity. This is the people that we are called to be. Not an oddity, not to stand out for the sake of standing out but different. Different only because the Light and love of Jesus Chris shines so perfectly through us that others can't help but notice. Then others will cry out, " You got to see this," and it will be for the right reasons.

Chapter Twenty Six

HOW MAY I SERVE YOU?

"Your meal is ready sir," the waiter had said. As I turned from my conversation with my friend, my breath was taken away. It was beautiful, no, magnificent. There before me on a cream colored platter with gold trim was one of my favorite dishes. It was called Cappa Gallo. It consisted of large gulf coast shrimp, scallops, bacon pieces, sundried tomatoes, red and green bellpepper, onions sautéed in whipping cream which makes a heavenly white sauce. This was served over a bed of angel hair pasta. A slice of orange with a garnish of sprouts trimmed out the plate. A large fresh cut salad with blue cheese dressing and real blue cheese crumbled on it sat next to a basket of homemade yeast rolls. It was a touch of heaven. "I could live in a place like this," I thought. As the waiter returned with a large glass of sweet tea and a dish of blackberry cobbler topped with ice cream, my cell phone rang.

Finding out that I had to leave immediately, I asked the waiter to put these items in a to-go bag for me, so I could enjoy them later. When he returned, I quickly paid, grabbed the bag from his hand and rushed of the handle the crisis.

Several hours later time and situation allowed me to take the time to enjoy the meal I had relished so much. As I was about to dine a close friend came in. I was excited to share this feast with him, I had often told him about what a wonderful dining experience was to be had, and he had promised to try it some time with me. This couldn't have worked out better. Setting the table my friend quickly tore into the bag in preparation to help dish out the meal. "Ugh…" he cried as he covered his hand with his mouth, trying to suppress his nausea. In horror I took the bag and looked inside.

There to my dismay I realized what the server at the restaurant had done. Instead of properly packaging the food, he simply poured the contents of each dish into the plastic lined bag, the main course, the salad, the rolls, pie ice-cream and tea now all swirled around together resembling something that someone else had already tried to digest and couldn't contain. It was horrible, why would anyone have wanted to have that in the first place I thought.

your clothes. And I promise I have even on several occasions see their yellow eyes staring down at me as they taunted me calling out who, who ,who….

Well anyway that leads to the problem that I have today. You see when I came home from work this afternoon, you guessed it. One of those trees had managed to slip into my house and hide it's self in the corner of the living room by the fireplace. Now I know that a few years ago we bought a fake one so that we wouldn't have to run the risk of one getting in the house. But somehow this giant evergreen has managed a coup. And taken over part of the house. Demanding that if it isn't fed a fresh supply of wrapped packages daily it will come into my room one night and I will wake up root bound or something. Anyway that is why I am writing you. After a quick look at my budget I am afraid that I may not be able to feed it new gifts fast enough. So I thought that I would let you know my circumstance so that if you had anything left over that your tree didn't demand you might like top pass it on to me so I can put it under mine. A chainsaw would be great. Oh, well it was just a thought…..

Chapter Twenty Nine

"CHRISTMAS REVIVAL"

T'was the night before Christmas, And all through God's house.

Excitement was building; the special services were all planned out.

As the people all arrived, and the programs were given.

The prayer rooms were filled, With Saints calling on heaven.

For what greater gift could we give,

Than to offer to Christ a new life to give?

Through all the practices and dedication,

We must remember our own consecration.

For in all this festive atmosphere,

We might forget why we are truly here.

You see a child was born in a stable one time,

To give New Hope to lives like yours and mine.

So when we gather to celebrate the Messiah's arrival,

What could be better than a Christmas revival.

About the Author

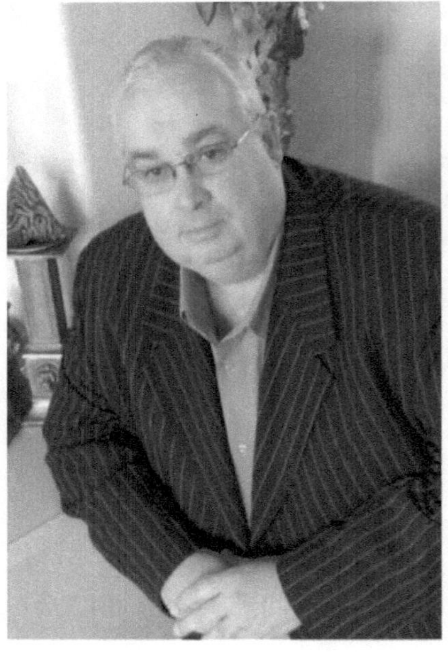

Greg Bullock is Lives in Lake Dallas Texas and works as an Electrical Design Engineering Specialist working with Heavy Industrial Electrical applications. In His free time He is involved in the different ministry works associated with "The Pentecostals of Katy Texas" and "The Pentecostals of Lewisville Texas". He is one of the Staff Ministers, Sunday School Teachers, Small Group Leaders, and Music ministers currently at the Lewisville campus. His free time is divided between his many different hobbies. He enjoys writing, playing music, creating both pen & Ink and oil paintings, building guitars and long Jeep rides

Acknowledgments

Greg has been married to his "Wonderful Wife" Kay for over 43 years and admits he would be completely lost without her. Greg would be quick to tell you that without her in his life he would not have accomplished anything. In August of 1974 Kay introduced Greg to Jesus and his life has been forever changed. A young man then with no purpose in his life found the compass he his life by and his life's course was forever changed.

In 2010 Greg & Kay moved to Katy Texas and combined their ministry efforts with those of Rev. Robert L. and Shara McKee as a part of "The Pentecostals of Katy". Working under the direction and encouragement of the McKee's ministry has allowed them to believe in and grow their ministries into directions that never seemed possible before, and for that they will forever be grateful. On many occasions both Rob and Shara have encouraged Greg to write these stories down and so without them this book may not exist today.

MON AMI LE MEURTRIER
Par A. Conan Doyle

«Le numéro 481 n'est pas meilleur, docteur», dit le gardien en chef avec un accent légèrement réprobateur, en regardant par le coin de ma porte.

"Confound 481", ai-je répondu derrière les pages de l' *Australian Sketcher* .

« Et 61 ans dit que ses trompes lui font mal. Tu ne pourrais rien faire pour lui ?

«C'est une pharmacie ambulante», dis-je. «Il a en lui toute la pharmacopée britannique. Je crois que ses tubes sont aussi sains que les vôtres.

« Ensuite, il y a le 7 et le 108, ils sont chroniques », poursuit le gardien en jetant un coup d'œil sur un bout de papier bleu. « Et 28 personnes ont arrêté leur travail hier – il a dit que soulever des objets lui avait donné un point de suture sur le côté. Je veux que vous jetiez un œil à lui, si cela ne vous dérange pas, docteur. Il y en a 81 aussi – celui qui a tué John Adamson dans le brick Corinthian – il s'est comporté horriblement pendant la nuit, criant et criant, il l'a fait, et rien ne l'a arrêté non plus.

"Très bien, je le verrai plus tard", dis-je en jetant négligemment mon papier et en me versant une tasse de café. « Rien d'autre à signaler, je suppose, gardien ?

Le fonctionnaire sortit la tête un peu plus loin dans la pièce. "Je vous demande pardon, docteur", dit-il sur un ton confidentiel, "mais je remarque que 82 est un peu enrhumé, et ce serait peut-être une bonne excuse pour que vous lui rendiez visite et discutiez."

La tasse de café s'arrêta à mi-chemin de mes lèvres alors que je regardais avec étonnement le visage sérieux de l'homme.

"Une excuse?" J'ai dit. "Une excuse? De quoi parlez-vous, McPherson ? Vous me voyez marcher toute la journée dans mon cabinet , quand je ne m'occupe pas des prisonniers, et revenir chaque soir fatigué comme un chien, et vous parlez de trouver une excuse pour faire plus de travail.

« Vous l'aimeriez, docteur », dit le directeur McPherson en insinuant l'une de ses épaules dans la pièce. « L'histoire de cet homme vaut la peine d'être écoutée si vous parvenez à l'amener à la raconter, même s'il n'est pas ce qu'on appellerait libre dans son discours. Peut-être que vous ne savez pas qui est 82 ?

"Non, je ne m'en soucie pas, et je m'en fiche non plus", répondis-je, convaincu qu'un voyou local était sur le point de m'imposer comme une célébrité.

« C'est Maloney, dit le gardien, celui qui a servi de preuve à Queen après les meurtres de Bluemansdyke .

"Tu ne le dis pas?" J'ai éjaculé en posant ma tasse avec étonnement. J'avais entendu parler de cette horrible série de meurtres et j'en avais lu un récit dans un magazine londonien bien avant de mettre les pieds dans la colonie. Je me souvenais que les atrocités commises avaient complètement occulté les crimes de Burke et Hare, et que l'un des plus crapuleux de la bande avait sauvé sa peau en trahissant ses compagnons. "Es-tu sûr?" J'ai demandé.

« Oh, oui, c'est bien lui, c'est vrai. Faites-le ressortir un peu et il vous étonnera. C'est un homme à connaître, c'est Maloney ; c'est-à-dire avec modération ; et la tête a souri, s'est agitée et a disparu, me laissant finir mon petit-déjeuner et ruminer ce que j'avais entendu.

Le poste de chirurgien dans une prison australienne n'est pas une position enviable. Cela peut être supportable à Melbourne ou à Sydney, mais la petite ville de Perth a peu d'attractions à recommander, et ces quelques-unes sont épuisées depuis longtemps. Le climat était détestable et la société loin d'être agréable. Les moutons et les bovins constituaient le soutien de

« Vous avez la loi de votre côté », dit le gouverneur ; « Nous ne vous retiendrons donc plus. Faites-lui sortir, gardien.

Il l'aurait fait aussi, le méchant au cœur noir, si je n'avais pas mendié, prié et proposé de payer pour ma nourriture et mon logement, ce qui est plus que ce qu'aucun prisonnier n'a jamais fait avant moi. Il m'a laissé rester à ces conditions ; et pendant trois mois j'ai été enfermé là-haut avec tous les larrikin du township qui criaient de l'autre côté du mur. C'était un joli traitement pour un homme qui avait servi son pays !

Enfin, un matin, le gouverneur revint.

"Eh bien, Maloney," dit-il, "combien de temps vas-tu nous honorer de ta société ?"

J'aurais pu planter un couteau dans son corps maudit, et je l'aurais fait aussi si nous avions été seuls dans la brousse ; mais je dus sourire, le caresser et le flatter, car je craignais qu'il ne me fasse renvoyer.

« Vous êtes un coquin infernal, dit-il ; telles étaient ses paroles, adressées à un homme qui l'avait aidé autant qu'il savait. « Mais je ne veux pas d'une justice brutale ici ; et je pense que je vois le moyen de te faire sortir de Dunedin.

« Je ne vous oublierai jamais, gouverneur, dis-je ; « et, par Dieu ! Je ne le ferai jamais."

«Je ne veux ni de vos remerciements ni de votre gratitude», répondit-il; ce n'est pas pour vous que je le fais, mais simplement pour maintenir l'ordre dans la ville. Il y a un bateau à vapeur qui part demain de West Quay pour Melbourne, et nous vous ferons monter à bord. Elle est annoncée à cinq heures du matin, alors préparez-vous.

J'ai emballé le peu de choses que j'avais et j'ai été sorti clandestinement par une porte dérobée, juste avant l'aube. Je me suis dépêché, j'ai pris mon billet au nom d'Isaac Smith et je suis monté sain et sauf à bord du bateau de Melbourne. Je me souviens avoir entendu sa vis grincer dans l'eau alors que les funes étaient larguées, et avoir regardé les lumières de Dunedin alors que je m'appuyais sur les pavois, avec la pensée agréable que je les laissais derrière moi pour toujours. Il me semblait qu'un monde nouveau était devant moi et que tous mes ennuis avaient été écartés. Je suis descendu en bas et j'ai pris un café, et je suis remonté en me sentant mieux que depuis le matin où je me suis réveillé pour trouver ce maudit Irlandais qui m'avait emmené debout au-dessus de moi avec un six coups.

Le jour s'était alors levé et nous naviguions le long de la côte, bien hors de vue de Dunedin. J'ai flâné pendant quelques heures et, lorsque le soleil s'est levé, d'autres passagers sont montés sur le pont et m'ont rejoint. L'un d'eux, un type un peu gai, m'a regardé longuement, puis est venu et a commencé à parler.

"L'exploitation minière, je suppose?" dit-il.

"Oui", dis-je.

« Vous avez fait votre pile ? » il demande.

« Assez juste », dis-je.

«J'y étais moi-même», dit-il; « J'ai travaillé aux champs de Nelson pendant trois mois et j'ai dépensé tout ce que je gagnais pour acheter une concession salée qui s'est effondrée le deuxième jour. Cependant, j'y suis retourné et je suis devenu riche ; mais quand le chariot d'or descendait vers les colonies, il a été bloqué par ces maudits rangers, et il ne restait plus un centime rouge.

«C'était un mauvais travail», dis-je.

« M'a brisé, m'a ruiné. Qu'à cela ne tienne, je les ai tous vus pendus pour cela ; cela le rend plus facile à supporter. Il n'en reste qu'un : le méchant qui a témoigné. Je mourrais heureux si je pouvais le rencontrer. Il y a deux choses que je dois faire si je le rencontre.

"Qu'est ce que c'est?" dis-je négligemment.

dans une sorte de marais, à plusieurs milles à l'est de Londres. J'étais trempé et à moitié mort de faim, mais je me suis rendu péniblement en ville, j'ai acheté un nouveau matériel dans un magasin de déchets et, après avoir dîné, j'ai pris un lit dans le logement le plus calme que j'ai pu trouver.

Je me suis réveillé assez tôt – une habitude que l'on prend dans la brousse – et heureusement pour moi, je l'ai fait. La toute première chose que j'ai vue en jetant un coup d'œil par une fente du volet, c'est un de ces policiers infernaux qui se tenaient juste en face et regardaient les fenêtres. Il n'avait pas d'épaulettes ni d'épée, comme nos pièges, mais il y avait quand même une sorte d'air de famille, et la même expression de occupé. Qu'ils m'aient suivi tout le temps, ou si la femme qui m'a loué le lit n'aimait pas mon apparence, c'est plus que je n'ai jamais pu découvrir. Il est apparu alors que je le regardais et a noté l'adresse de la maison dans un livre. J'avais peur qu'il sonne à la cloche, mais je suppose que ses ordres étaient simplement de me surveiller, car après avoir encore regardé attentivement les fenêtres, il s'est éloigné dans la rue.

J'ai compris que ma seule chance était d'agir immédiatement. J'ai enfilé mes vêtements, j'ai ouvert doucement la fenêtre et, après m'être assuré qu'il n'y avait personne, je me suis laissé tomber par terre et j'ai couru de toutes mes forces. J'avais parcouru deux ou trois milles lorsque le vent m'a lâché ; et comme j'ai vu un grand bâtiment avec des gens qui entraient et sortaient, j'y suis entré aussi et j'ai découvert que c'était une gare. Un train partait justement pour Douvres pour rencontrer le bateau français, alors j'ai pris un billet et j'ai sauté dans une voiture de troisième classe.

Il y avait quelques autres types dans la voiture, tous deux de jeunes mendiants à l'air innocent. Ils ont commencé à parler de ceci et de cela, tandis que j'étais assis tranquillement dans un coin et j'écoutais. Ensuite, ils ont commencé par l'Angleterre et les pays étrangers, et ainsi de suite. Écoutez, docteur, c'est un fait. L'un d'eux commence à s'interroger sur la justice des lois anglaises. « Tout est juste et honnête », dit-il ; « Il n'y a pas de police secrète, ni d'espionnage, comme à l'étranger », et bien d'autres choses du même genre . C'était plutôt dur avec moi, n'est-ce pas, d'écouter ce foutu jeune imbécile , avec la police qui me suivait comme mon ombre ?

Je suis arrivé à Paris tout de suite, j'y ai changé une partie de mon or, et pendant quelques jours j'ai cru que je m'en étais débarrassé, et j'ai commencé à songer à m'installer pour un peu de repos. J'en avais besoin à ce moment-là, car je ressemblais plus à un fantôme qu'à un homme. Vous n'avez jamais été poursuivi par la police, je suppose ? Eh bien, vous n'avez pas besoin d'avoir l'air offensé, je ne voulais pas de mal. Si jamais vous en aviez eu, vous sauriez que cela dépérit un homme comme un mouton atteint de pourriture.

Un soir, je suis allé à l'Opéra et j'en ai pris une loge, car j'étais très rouge. Je sortais entre les actes lorsque j'ai rencontré un type qui se prélassait dans le couloir. La lumière tomba sur son visage et je vis que c'était le mud-pilot qui nous avait embarqués dans la Tamise. Sa barbe avait disparu, mais j'ai reconnu l'homme d'un seul coup d'œil, car j'ai une bonne mémoire des visages.

Je vous le dis, docteur, je me suis senti désespéré un instant. J'aurais pu le poignarder si nous avions été seuls, mais il me connaissait assez bien pour ne jamais m'en laisser l'occasion. C'était plus que je ne pouvais supporter plus longtemps, alors je me suis approché de lui et je l'ai tiré à l'écart, là où nous serions libres de tous les transats et des spectateurs du théâtre.

"Combien de temps vas-tu continuer comme ça ?" Je lui ai demandé.

Il parut un peu troublé pendant un moment, mais ensuite il comprit qu'il ne servait à rien de tourner autour du pot, alors il répondit sans détour :

"Jusqu'à ce que tu retournes en Australie", dit-il.

« Ne savez-vous pas, dis-je, que j'ai servi le gouvernement et obtenu une grâce gratuite ?

क्रम-सूची

प्रश्न बन कर खड़ा है, जिसने हमारे अन्तर्मन को ही बिलकुल शुष्क बना दिया है | नतीजतन संवेदनहीनता और असुरक्षा की भावना हमारे अंदर घर करती जा रही है ।संग्रह की कहानियों को पढ़ कर ऐसा लगता है कि कथा लेखिका इन सारी बातों से अच्छी तरह वाकिफ हैं और उनकी यह कोशिश है कि वे इन विसंगतियों के प्रति अपना रोष अपनी कहानियों के माध्यम से व्यक्त करें और उसमे वे सफल भी हुई हैं ।

डॉ. सोनिया गुप्ता की कहानियाँ भले ही आकार में छोटी हों पर उनका कैनवास बहुत बड़ा है और वे पाठक को प्रभावित करने मे सक्षम हैं , उनके इस कहानी संग्रह से उनके कथा सामर्थ्य का सुंदर परिचय मिलता है । कहानियाँ रोचक, दिल के कोमल से रेशे को स्पर्श करने वाली , और एक ख़ास संदेश को दर्शाती हुई नजर आती हैं । इसमें कोई दो राय नहीं कि डॉ. सोनिया का कथाकार मन समाज की विसंगतियों ,उसकी चिंताओं और व्याप्त कुरीतियों को देख कर या महसूस करके असहज होता है, जिसे वह कथा के माध्यम से प्रस्तुत कर इससे निजात पाने की सहज कोशिश करता है और उसमे वह सफल भी होता है । इनकी कहानियों को पढ़ कर ऐसा लगता है मानो कथाकार को कैमरे की भाषा की बखूबी समझ हो और वह लॉन्ग शॉट तथा क्लोज अप शॉट की तरह कहानी के किरदारों को भी सामने लाता है ताकि कही गई बात का पूरा असर हो सके।डॉ. सोनिया गुप्ता की कहानियों मे शिल्प और विषय दोनों ही दृष्टि से कोई पुनरावृति नहीं नज़र आती । मैं डॉ. सोनिया को उनके इस पहले कहानी संग्रह के लिए बहुत बहुत बधाई देता हूँ और मुझे पूरा विश्वास है कि इनके पूर्व प्रकाशित काव्य संग्रहों कि भांति इसका भी अवश्य स्वागत होगा और इस संग्रह की हर कहानी पाठकों को सोचने पर विवश करेगी |

☙

इन्हीं शुभकामनाओं के साथ-

- राजेश कुमार सिन्हा

- वर्तमान पता : फ्लैट संख्या -5,प्लॉट संख्या -116, सुखदाई सी एच एस, एस वी रोड, खार (वेस्ट),मुंबई -400052
- मोबाइल : 7506345031

आभार

❧

कहते हैं कि हर इंसान की सफलता के पीछे किसी न किसी का प्रत्यक्ष या अप्रत्यक्ष रूप में सहयोग अवश्य होता है और ऐसे व्यक्ति विशेष का शब्दों में आभार व्यक्त करना इतना सरल नहीं होता, पर फिर भी इस छोटे से शब्द 'आभार' में बहुत गहरा भेद छिपा होता है | मैं पेशे से एक दंत चिकित्स्क हूँ, और मैंने स्वप्न में भी नहीं सोचा था कभी कि एक दिन मुझे लेखिका/कवयित्री बनने का सौभाग्य भी प्राप्त होगा | मेरा यह साहित्यिक सफ़र बहुत अनोखा रहा जिसमें बहुत से लोगों का आशीष रहा |

सर्वप्रथम शब्दों और ज्ञान की देवी "माँ सरस्वती जी" का आभार, जिन्होंने मेरे साधारण से शब्दों को भावपूर्ण माला में पिरो दिया |

कोटि कोटि नमन मेरे पूजनीय माता पिता को, जिन्होंने मुझे जन्म दिया और किसी काबिल बनाया | आज मेरे पिताश्री इस नश्वर संसार में जीवित नहीं,पर उनकी सिखाई हर सीख आज तक मुझे प्रेरणा देती है | मेरी माँ ने मेरे हर प्रतिकूल और अनुकूल समय में मेरा साथ दिया|

प्रभु और माता पिता समान मेरे सभी शिक्षकों का हार्दिक आभार जिन्होंने मेरी पढ़ाई के साथ साथ मेरे हुनर को भी सराहा |

शत शत नमन मेरे परम् आदरणीय साहित्यिक गुरुदेव श्री लव कुमार 'प्रणय' जी का, जिनका आशीष हमेशा मुझपर रहा |

उन सभी गुरुजनों का आभार, जिन्होंने मुझे साहित्य जगत में एक पहचान दी |

मेरा विशेष आभार आदरणीय सर 'राजेश कुमार सिन्हा जी' को, जिन्होंने अपना कीमती समय निकालकर मेरी कहानियों को पढ़ा और मार्गदर्शन किया, तथा इस पुस्तक की सुंदर सी भूमिका भी लिखी |आप एक अच्छे कवि और लेखक ही नहीं अपितु, एक अच्छे इंसान भी हैं, जो हमेशा दूसरों को प्रोत्साहित करते हैं | आपके

1
अप्रितम भावना

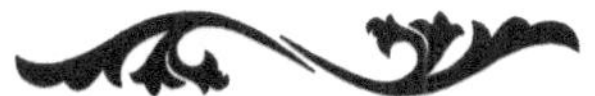

वो रोज सुबह गुब्बारों, खिलौनों से लदा अपना वही पुराना ठेला लेकर आता था, और बैठ जाता था उसी हरे भरे नीम के पेड़ तले | बुजुर्ग अधेड़ उम्र का शरीर, पर चेहरे पर रौनक और उमंग ऐसी, कि किसी नवयुवक की भी न होगी | छोटे छोटे बच्चे सब उसके आते ही घेर लेते उसके ठेले को | अनोखी बात यह भी थी कि वह हर बच्चे को खिलौनों के साथ एक उपहार मुफ़्त में बाँटता था |

कोई नहीं जानता था, वो बूढ़ा व्यक्ति कहाँ से आता था, क्यूँकि गाँव में तो उसे किसी ने देखा नहीं था | सबको बड़ी जिज्ञासा थी उस बूढ़े व्यक्ति के बारे में जानने की | एक दिन अचानक एक बच्चे ने उनसे यह प्रश्न पूछ ही डाला "बाबा ये आप इतनी अधेड़ उम्र में भी इतना परिश्रम कर रहे हैं, क्या घर में कोई तंगी है आपके? क्या आपकी औलाद नहीं है ?" बाबा मुस्करा उठे और चुप रहे | तभी अचानक उनका मोबाईल बजा | उन्हें आवाज़ सुनाई नहीं दे रही थी साफ़, तो उन्होंने स्पीकर ऑन कर लिया और बात करने लगे |

"और भई, प्रोफेसर साहब कैसे हैं आप" ? किसी ने उनसे पूछा | बात होती रही, ख़त्म होते ही बाबा ने फ़ोन रखा |

बच्चा उनकी बातें सुनकर दंग रह गया |

प्रोफेसर ? "आप प्रोफेसर हैं बाबा" | बच्चा बोला |

3

कुदरत का करिश्मा

सतीश एक ग़रीब किसान था | उसकी तीन बेटियां और एक बेटा था | उसने अपना सब कुछ लुटाकर अपने बच्चों की पढ़ाई लिखाई पर ही अपना सारा जीवन बिता दिया |

सतीश को अपने बच्चों के भविष्य की चिंता रहती थी | कैसे तीन बेटियों की शादी करेगा वो? कहाँ से मिल पाएँगे उपयुक्त वर उसकी तीनों बेटियों के लिए ? उसकी पत्नी सुषमा हमेशा उसको होंसला देती "सब ईश्वर पर छोड़ दीजिये, वो स्वयं रास्ता बनाता है सबका" |

वक़्त बीतता गया | सतीश के तीनों बच्चे बड़े हो गए और उनकी मेहनत रंग लाई | बेटा, लॉ की पढ़ाई करके वकील बन गया और एक बेटी डॉक्टर तथा दो बेटियां इंजीनियर बनी | अब उनके विवाह की चिंता | सतीश जगह जगह इश्तिहार देता, पर कहीं से कोई जवाब न आता| सतीश की डॉक्टर बेटी 'मानवी', सांवली थी, इतना पढ़ लिख कर भी उसका हाथ मांगने को कोई तैयार न होता | सतीश हताश हो गया था, जब तक बड़ी बेटी का विवाह न करेगा, तब तक दोनों भी नहीं करेंगी | बेटा तो चलो अभी छोटा है |

एक दिन मानवी को बाहर किसी शहर में जाना पड़ा, जहाँ एक महामारी फ़ैल गयी और बहुत लोग बीमार पड़ गए | लाख कोशिश की, किसी डॉक्टर ने उस महामारी में कोई योगदान नहीं दिया | पर मानवी ने साहस दिखाया और सबका ईलाज करने को तैयार हुई | उस महामारी का शिकार शहर के मुख्यमंत्री का परिवार भी

बना | मानवी ने उनकी अच्छे से देखभाल की और उनको पुनः स्वस्थ कर दिया | मुख्यमंत्री ने उसका आभार व्यक्त किया और उसको अपने घर आमंत्रित किया |

मानवी उनके घर गयी और वहां सबको वो बहुत पसंद आई | मुख्यमंत्री का एक बेटा था 'किशोर', जो कि विदेश में एक बड़ा व्यापारी था | उन्होंने अपने बेटे के लिए मानवी का हाथ माँगा | मानवी को यकीन ही नहीं हो रहा था ये सब सुनकर | उसने बोला कि वो अपने माता पिता से अनुमति लिए बग़ैर ये रिश्ता नहीं कर सकती | मुख्यमंत्री ने बोला, हाँ उनकी आज्ञा तो आवश्यक है, तुम उनको फोन करो और सारी बात स्पष्ट बताओ, फिर हम उनसे मिलने जाएंगे |

मानवी ने घर फोन किया और अपने पापा को सब बताया | वो बहुत ख़ुश हो गए और मिलने का समय निश्चित कर लिया |

मुख्यमंत्री और उनकी पत्नी मानवी के परिवार से मिलने गए | और वहां उन्होंने अपने बेटे के लिए मानवी का हाथ माँगा | सतीश सोच रहा था कि हम इतने छोटे घराने के लोग और ये इतने बड़े, क्या निभा पाएंगे ? सतीश को सोच में देखकर मुख्यमंत्री एक दम बोले "आप बेकार सोच रहे हैं सतीश जी, रिश्ते छोटे बड़े नहीं होते, वे तो प्रेम और आदर से बनते हैं | आपकी बेटी ने जो हमारे परिवार के लिए किया, वो कोई और नहीं कर सकता था | अब तो बस विवाह की तैयारी कीजिये, हमारा बेटा परसों ही आ रहा है विदेश से | आकर मानवी को साथ ले जाएगा और मानवी का जीवन भी उज्ज्वल बनेगा वहां जाकर" | सतीश की आँखों से ख़ुशी के अश्रु बहने लगे |

मानवी का विवाह बड़े हर्ष उल्लास से सम्पन्न हुआ और वह हँसी ख़ुशी अपने परिवार में घुल मिल गयी | सतीश के मन से बहुत बड़ा बोझ उतर गया, चलो एक बेटी का तो विवाह हुआ | बाकी भी भगवान करेंगे कुछ हल | दिन बीतते गए | मानवी विदेश में रहने लगी |

एक दिन उसके पति ने उसको बोला कि मेरे दो बहुत घनिष्ठ मित्र हैं, यहीं रहते हैं हमारे से थोड़ा दूर, क्यों न तुम्हारी बहनों के लिए उनकी बात चलाएं , कैसा रहेगा ? सब एक साथ यहां रहेंगे, तुम्हें भी अपना सा लगेगा |

बहुत चलेगा भाभी जी" और वो चला गया "अच्छा चलता हूँ, आप आराम कीजिये"|

थोड़ी देर बाद, माया के दिमाग में उस आदमी की बात आयी "क्यों न उसकी बात पर अम्ल करूँ ?"उसने सोचा एक टिफिन सिस्टम से शुरू करती हूँ |

माया ने उसी दिन से अपना टिफिन का काम शुरू किया | और धीरे धीरे उसका काम बढ़ता गया, उसके खाने की सब तारीफ़ करते थे | एक दिन माया मुकेश को मिलने अस्पताल जाने लगी, तो कोई विदेश से आया हुआ बड़ा बिजनेसमैन उनके घर आया |

"जी नमस्ते, वो तो अभी घर पर नहीं ", माया बोली |

"हम उनसे नहीं, आपसे मिलने आये हैं माया जी, बहुत तारीफ सुनी है आपके खाने की, हम यहां एक रेस्टोरेंट खोलना चाहते हैं, जिसमें आपको मैनेजर बनाने का निर्णय लिया हमने"

माया दंग रह गयी "जी पर मैं ?"

"आप बिलकुल निश्चिंत रहिये, हम आपको पूरा सहयोग देंगे", उसने माया से बोला |

माया ने कहा "मुझे अपने पति से इस बारे में अनुमति लेनी पड़ेगी" |

उसने बोला, चलिए अभी चलते हैं, साथ ही |दोनों अस्पताल पहुंचे, और मुकेश को सारी बात बताई | मुकेश बहुत खुश हुआ और मान गया| माया ने कॉन्ट्रैक्ट साइन किया और उस दिन से उनके अच्छे दिनों की शुरुवात होने लगी | माया का काम बहुत अच्छा चला और उधर मुकेश भी स्वस्थ होने लगा | माया ने मुकेश से बोला "देखा, मैंने कहा था न सब ठीक हो जाएगा"|

आज माया के अपने खुद के कितने होटल हैं, जिनमें कितने ही कर्मचारी काम करते हैं | उन्होंने सारा पिछला कर्जा चुका दिया और दीर्घ समय पश्चात वे थोड़ी ख़ुशी के पल जी रहे हैं|

6

छल का जाल

निखिल भोला भाला सा लड़का था, अपने गाँव में सबका चहेता | उसकी आयु केवल १० बरस की थी | उसकी बचपन से इच्छा थी की वो मुंबई जाकर फिल्मों में काम करे, पर गाँव में कौन उसका साथ देता | बस इस ख़्वाब को वो अपनी आँखों में सजाये रहता | अकसर वो अपने दोस्तों के साथ खेल खेल में हीरो का रोल करता, उनके साथ फिल्म की तरह काम करता | बड़ा मायूस होता था वो ये सोचकर कि कब उसका यह ख़्वाब हक़ीक़त में बदलेगा |

एक दिन, वो अपने गाँव के कुँए के पास बैठा, फ़िल्मी हीरो की तरह एक्टिंग कर रहा था, अकेला ही | अचानक वहां एक अनजान सा व्यक्ति आया, उसने मुंह पर नकाब ओढ़ रखा था | उसने निखिल को देखकर उसके पास जाकर बोला "हीरो बनेगा, क्या?"

निखिल एक दम कूद पड़ा, "हाँ चाचा, मैं मुंबई जाना चाहता हूँ, फिल्मों में काम करना चाहता हूँ" |

"मैं मुंबई से ही आया हूँ, चलेगा मेरे साथ मुंबई, मैं ले जाऊँगा तुझे" वो आदमी बोला

"हाँ चाचा, ले जाओ न मुझे"

"पर तेरे माँ बापू भेज देंगे तुझे ?"

"नहीं, वो तो नहीं भेजेंगे"

8

आदमी बने रहने का ढोंग

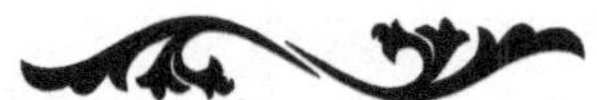

कविता के माँ बाप बचपन में ही गुज़र गए थे | उसकी एक छोटी बहन थी 'ममता' और एक छोटा भाई 'मनोज' | कविता घर में सबसे बड़ी थी, घर की ज़िम्मेदारी उसी के कंधों पर थी सारी | वे वैसे ही ग़रीब घर से थे | घर का गुज़ारा बड़ी मुश्किल से होता था | कविता कपड़े सिलकर पैसे कमाती थी | उसकी बहन ममता उसका हाथ बँटाती और घर के काम में उसकी मदद करती थी | पर उनका भाई मनोज कोई काम नहीं करता था और वो बुरी संगत में पड़ गया | जो भी पैसे उसकी बहनें एकत्र करतीं, वो चोरी करके जुए में उड़ा देता | जब वो देने से मना करती, तो उनपर हाथ तक उठा देता था | कविता और उसकी बहन मज़बूर थी | कुछ नहीं कर सकती थी, बस रोज़ भगवान से प्रार्थना करती रहती कि उनके भाई को सदबुद्धि दे |

एक दिन, मनोज सारे पैसे जुए में हार गया, अब कुछ न बचा उसके पास |

घर पहुँचा तो अचानक कविता को अचम्भा सा हुआ, जब उसके कानों में एक ध्वनि सुनाई दी " प्यारी बहना, कहाँ हो तुम ? देखो मैं क्या लाया तुम्हारे और ममता के लिए"| कविता को लगा मानो कोई वहम हुआ हो उसको | ममता भी देखकर चकित हो रही थी | ममता रसोई में चाय बनाने लगी, मनोज ने उसके हाथ से बर्तन पकड़ लिए और बोला "आज चाय मैं बनाऊँगा, तुम आराम करो" | मनोज ने चाय बनाई और उन दोनों को परोसी | दोनों को समझ नहीं आ रहा था आखिर क्या माजरा है |

"बहना, मुझे माफ़ कर दो, मैंने तुम दोनों को बहुत परेशान किया आज तक, बस अब नहीं, अब तुम काम नहीं करोगी, अब मैं तुम्हारे सारे दुःख दूर कर दूँगा | मेरी आँखों पर से पट्टी उतर गयी है और मुझे अकल आ गयी है" | वो उनसे दावा करने लगा कि आज के बाद कभी बुरी संगत नहीं अपनाएगा और घर की तरफ़ ध्यान देगा |

कविता पहले तो थोड़ा सोच विचार में पड़ गयी, परन्तु नारी होती ही कोमल हृदय धर्ता और सहनशीलता की मूरत है | उसने भाई की बातों पर यकीन कर लिया और ख़ुशी से झूम उठी |

थोड़ी देर बाद मनोज ने कविता को बातों में फिसला कर उससे कुछ पैसे मांगे यह कहकर कि वो कल से एक नया काम शुरू करेगा | कविता स्नेहवश आकर भाई की बातों को सच मान लेती है और झट से पैसे दे देती है | "ठीक है भाई, अच्छे से मन लगाकर काम करना, भगवान तुम्हें बहुत सफ़लता दे, यही कामना है हमारी" | कविता आरती की थाली लाई और तिलक लगाकर भाई की मंगलकामना की |

मनोज पैसे लेकर चला जाता है और फिर से जुए में उड़ा देता है, और कविता को रोज झूठ बोलकर निकल जाता है कि काम पर जा रहा है | सारे पैसे ऐसे ही व्यर्थ गँवा देता है | घर आकर वही बनावटी स्नेह दिखाता है अपनी बहनों को |

एक दिन कविता घर की सफ़ाई कर रही थी, कि अचानक दरवाजे पर आहट हुई " कोई है घर पर"? कविता जब बाहर गयी तो देखा पुलिस आई थी, उसके चेहरे का रंग उड़ गया | उसने कंपकपाते हुए पूछा "कहिये इंस्पेक्टर साहिब क्या बात है? किससे मिलना है आपको"?

"मनोज का घर यही है? इंस्पेक्टर ने पूछा |

कविता ने कहा "हांजी, यही है" |

"तुम्हारा क्या रिश्ता है उससे" ? इंस्पेक्टर ने पूछा |

"जी, मैं उनकी बहन हूँ, कविता " |

पुलिस चली गयी, और दूसरी जगह खोजने पर रामू उनके हाथ लग गया | पुलिस ने रामकृष्ण को बुलाया, और जानकर बहुत रोया वो | खेती बाड़ी करके अपना निर्वाह करता था | जैसे कैसे उसने रामू की जमानत करवा दी |

घर जाकर बहुत डांट लगाई उसको | मानो रामकृष्ण और उसकी पत्नी के सब अरमान बिखर गये हों |

अभी बेटी सुमन की शादी भी सर पर थी | क्या जवाब देंगे वे लड़के वालों को, डर के मारे सो नहीं पाए रात भर |

और वही डर सामने आ गया | सुबह होते ही, सुमन के ससुराल से संदेश आया, कि उन्होंने ये रिश्ता तोड़ दिया है | रामकृष्ण और उसका परिवार बिलख कर रह गया | दोनों बड़े दुखी हुए, अपनी सन्तान को ऐसा पाकर | पर फिर भी उनको रामू से आस थी, एक उम्मीद थी कि वो उनकी ममता की लाज रखेगा | जल्दी ही वो अपनी पढ़ाई करके वापिस आएगा |

कुछ समय बाद जब रामू वापिस आया, तो दोनों ने उसको सुमन के रिश्ते के बारे सब कुछ बताया | पर रामू का उत्तर सुनकर दोनों दंग रह गये | "ये कोई नई बात नहीं, माँ बापू, आजकल ये आम हो गया है, तो क्या हुआ, सुमन का रिश्ता कहीं और कर देना | मुझसे उम्मीद मत रखना, मेरे पास देने को कुछ नहीं | मेरा खुद का ही बहुत खर्चा है वहाँ" |

सुनकर और भी सदमे में चले गये दोनों | क्या ये वही अनाथ बालक है, जिसको हमने अपना नाम दिया, एक पहचान दी ? इसी दिन के लिए

दोनों की बरसों से बनाई एक 'आस की दहलीज' मानो आज टूट गयी |

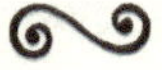

11

एक सीख जिसने ज़िंदगी बदल दी

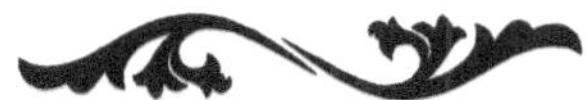

सरला रोज़ अपनी नौकरी पर जाया करती थी | कुछ दिनों से, घर वापिस आते हुए उसको एक आवाज़ सुनाई देती थी "अरे, भगवान के नाम पर दे दो बाबा, तुम्हारे बच्चे ख़ुश रहेंगे" एक नौजवान सी औरत साथ में बच्चे को लिए बैठी रहती थी फुटपाथ के किनारे और भीख मांगती रहती थी | सरला उसको कई दिन से देख रही थी, पर कुछ कहती नहीं थी | आज उस से रहा नहीं गया "ये क्यों तुम रोज़ ऐसे भीख मांगती रहती हो, और अपने बच्चे को भी यही सिखा रही हो, तुम्हारे पास तो चलता फिरता शरीर है, उसका उपयोग किसी काम में करो, ये लाचारी भरा जीवन जीना क्या तुम्हें अच्छा लगता है"?

"अरे मैडम जी, आप तो पैसे वाली हो, ये सब बोलना बहुत आसान है", वो औरत बोली |

"पैसा हर कोई कमाता है बहना, जैसे तुम यहां सुबह से बैठी हो, ऐसे ही हम भी सुबह से अपने घर से निकलते हैं, मेहनत करते हैं, तब जाकर ये पैसा एकत्र होता है, तुममें और मुझमें एक ही अंतर है, तुम अपना ईमान बेच कर पैसा कमा रही हो, पर मैं सम्मान से, और कोई अंतर् नहीं, दोनों इंसान हैं हम, दोनों के पास ये हाथ पांव हैं", बस ये बोला और सरला चली गयी |

उनके मुख से एक ही वाक्य निकला "मैं धनी हुआ बेटी तुझ जैसी पुत्री पाकर"|

रोते रोते अपनी बूढ़ी जुबान से वो बोलते रहे "क्या जिम्मेदारी निभाते हैं पुत्र ? दुनिया तरसती रह जाती है, एक बेटे को, पर क्या करना ऐसे बेटे का जिसको यह एहसास नहीं कि एक सन्तान का अपने माता पिता के प्रति क्या फर्ज़ होता है | जिन्दगी के एक मोड़ पर आकर शायद बेटे माँ बाप का तिरस्कार कर दें, परन्तु बेटियां ही हैं जो पराया धन होकर भी अपने माता पिता के प्रति हर फर्ज़ निभाती हैं, स्नेह लुटाती हैं | ऐसी होती हैं "बेटियां"|

हैरानी की बात यह है, इतना कुछ होकर भी कमला के भाई ने एक बार भी आकर कमला को आभार व्यक्त नहीं किया |

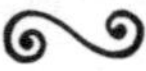

14

पराया अपना कहाँ बन सके

रघु और उसका मित्र राम कृष्ण रोज जाते थे उस ढाबे पर चाय का एक प्याला पीने, जहाँ वो बालक 'राजू' अपने नन्हें नन्हें हाथों से चाय बनाकर सब को परोसता था और झूठे बर्तन भी मांजता था | वे अकसर उसको देखा करते थे अपनी उम्र के उन बच्चों को निहारते हुए, जो पास ही की पाठशाला में पढ़ने आते थे | इच्छा उसकी भी बहुत होती थी कि वो भी उन सब की तरह अपने कंधों पर किताबों भरा बस्ता लाद कर, हाथों में कलम लेकर पढ़ लिख जाये और उन्नति करे |

जब भी वो सावन के महीने में अपने आस पास के बच्चों को पानी में किश्ती बहाते देखता, उसकी आँखों से अश्रु बहकर खुद ही इक मेघा बन जाते | वो तो शायद बचपन के मायने सीख ही न पाया, उसको तो यह बचपन शब्द सुन कर भी हँसी आती थी | बुढ़ापा क्या होता है, उसको यह एहसास अभी से होने लगा था | क्या कसूर था इस सब में उसका आखिर? क्या यही कि उसको गरीबी ने घेरे हुआ था या ये कि उसके सर पर माँ बाप का साया न था?

बहुत दिनों तक तो रघु और रामकृष्ण राजू के अंतर्मन की दशा का अवलोकन करते रहे, पर उनका खुद का हृदय दहक उठता था उसकी ये हालत देख कर | राम कृष्ण थोडा भावुक किस्म का इन्सान था | एक दिन राम कृष्ण ने रघु से पूछा कि क्यूँ न मैं इस बच्चे को आश्रय देकर अपना बना लूँ? राम कृष्ण अकेला था, बरसों गुजर गये उसकी पत्नी "शारदा" को इस दुनिया से गये |

'डॉक्टर है'

बड़ा आश्चर्य हुआ जानकर रश्मि को "डॉक्टर ?
    'पर कारण क्या रहा आपको बेघर करने का'?

"कुछ नहीं बेटी, बस मैंने एक दिन बहू को चाय बनाने को कह दिया, बेटे को गुस्सा आ गया कि मेरी पढ़ी लिखी पत्नी को घर का काम करने को कैसे कह दिया" |

बस और कुछ पूछने की हिम्मत न हुई रश्मि की | मन ही मन सोचने लगी "दुनिया कितनी बड़ी हो गई है, पर सोच आज भी छोटी, जो माँ-बाप संतान को किसी काबिल बनाते हैं, वही संतान एक ही पल में उन्हीं माता पिता को ठुकरा देती है, कैसी विडम्बना इस उन्नत समाज की? "

रश्मि ने उनसे कहा कि चलो मैं करती हूँ आपके पति का ईलाज, "मैं भी डॉक्टर हूँ"

'पर बेटी अभी ईलाज के लिए पैसे नहीं जुड़े'|

कोई बात नहीं माँ, बेटियाँ माँ-बाप से पैसे नहीं लेती, दुआएं लेती हैं | चलो अब देर न करो |

उनके पति को अस्पताल में दाखिल करवाया, और ईलाज शुरू कर दिया | धीरे धीरे उनका स्वास्थ्य सुधरने लगा | आज वे स्वस्थ हैं और रश्मि के साथ ही रहते हैं |

"भगवान ने हमें बेटे से भी बढ़कर ऐसी गुणवान बेटी दी है, हम तुम्हारे ऋणि रहेंगे सदैव बेटी", दोनों पति पत्नी ने रश्मि के सर पर हाथ रखकर दुआ दी |

"अरे माँ-बाबू जी, फिर से वही पराया न करिये" |

आज वे सभी एक परिवार की तरह एक साथ रहते हैं |

17

पहला उपवास

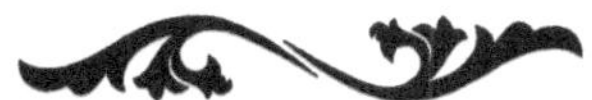

नेहा 7 बरस की थी, और वह बचपन से अपनी माँ को, नवरात्रों के उपवास रखते देखती आई थी, जिस से प्रेरित होकर, उसको भी उपवास रखने की प्रेरणा मिली |

इस बार नवरात्रे आए, तो उसने निर्णय लिया कि मैं भी उपवास रखूंगी, वो भी सारे | और उसे ये भी मालूम था कि उसकी माँ उसे ख़ूब डाँटेगी और बोलेगी "कोई उपवास नहीं रखना, बच्चे थोड़े अभी से रखते हैं उपवास" |

पर नेहा भी तो हठी थी | उसने पहले नवरात्रे की पूर्व रात्रि को अपनी माँ से बोला "मैं कल उपवास रखूंगी, और मुझे मना मत करना आप" | परन्तु माँ तो हो गयी गुस्सा "कोई उपवास नहीं रखना, समझ आ गयी?" पर नेहा सुनकर सो गयी |

सुबह उठते ही उसने एक योजना बनाई, माँ से बोला आज मेरा मन नहीं खाने का कुछ भी, माँ ने कहा 'मुझे पता है तू झूठ बोल रही है, तूने जरुर उपवास रखा होगा'

अरे नहीं माँ, आपने मना किया था, कैसे रखूंगी? फिर कुछ खा क्यूँ नहीं रही? माँ, खाऊँगी, पर अभी नहीं, अभी भूख नहीं, थोड़ी देर में खा लूँगी | चलो माँ मान गयी |

थोड़ी देर बाद फिर से बोलने लगी, 'चल खा ले, ये ले मैगी बनाई है, "अरे नहीं माँ, मेरे पेट में बहुत दर्द है आज, मुझे मैगी वैगी नहीं खानी | माँ मुझे वो चलाई की पट्टी खानी है, कहकर नेहा ने जिद्द की......

20
गरजते बादल

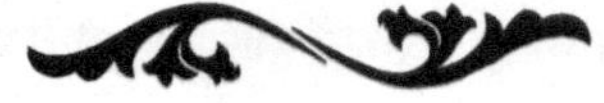

रामचंद्र एक गरीब किसान था | उसके तीन बच्चे थे "दो पुत्रियाँ और एक पुत्र" | रामचंद्र अपने घर में एकमात्र कमाई का साधन था | उसकी पत्नी, कमला उसके काम काज में उसकी मदद करती थी | वे सब एक सादा और खुशमय जीवन व्यतीत कर रहे थे |

एक दिन अचानक कमला चक्कर खाकर बेहोश हो गयी | रामचंद्र ने जैसे तैसे डॉक्टर को दिखाया | उसकी रिपोर्ट्स देखकर डॉक्टरों ने बताया कि कमला को कैंसर हो गया है, पर ख़तरे की बात नहीं, अभी उसका ईलाज हो सकता है | सुनते ही, रामचंद्र घबरा गया |

"डॉक्टर साहब, मेरी पत्नी का ईलाज कर दीजिये, इसके बिना मेरा कोई गुज़ारा नहीं, आज जो कुछ भी मैं थोड़ा बहुत कमाता हूँ, इसी की बदौलत"

"देखो, हम पूरी कोशिश करेंगे, पर खर्चा बहुत होगा इनके ईलाज में"|

"आप खर्च की फ़िक्र न करिये, मैं कोई न कोई इंतज़ाम कर लूंगा" |

डॉक्टरों ने कमला का ईलाज करने को हाँ भर दी और रामचंद्र को कुछ पैसे जमा करवाने को बोला |

रामचंद्र ने कहा "सरकार, अभी जितने हैं, आप ले लीजिये और इसका ईलाज शुरू कर दीजिये, बाकी मैं एकत्र करता हूँ "कहकर राम चंद्र चला गया |

अभी कमला साथ ही घर आयी थी "आप इतना इंतज़ाम कैसे करेंगे, रहने दीजिये मुझे, वैसे भी क्या करना है जी कर अब"

"चुप करो, ऐसी बातें तुम्हें शोभा नहीं देती, मैं हूँ न, करता हूँ कुछ, तुम बस आराम करो"

रामचंद्र कमला को बिस्तर पर लिटाकर बाहर चला गया | उनकी दोनों बेटियों ने घर संभाला और बेटा खेती बाड़ी में रामचंद्र का हाथ बंटाता |

रामचंद्र को समझ नहीं आ रहा था क्या करे, बैठा रहा, सोचता रहा कुछ देर, फिर उसने सोचा, क्यों न सरपंच से उधार ले आए कुछ पैसे और फिर वापिस कर देगा | दौड़े दौड़े सरपंच से मिलने गया और उसको सारा हाल बताया |

'सरपंच जी मुझे आपकी मदद चाहिए, कुछ पैसे उधार, अपनी पत्नी के ईलाज के लिए'

"पर तुम्हें सूत समेत लौटाने होंगे" सरपंच बोला|

"जी हाँ, पक्का वायदा"

सरपंच ने रामचंद्र को पैसे दिए और उसने डॉक्टरों को जमा करवा दिए "लीजिये डॉक्टर साहिब, अब जल्दी से मेरी पत्नी का ईलाज शुरू कर दीजिये"

रामचंद्र उस दिन से अपने खेत में दिन रात काम करने लगा, उसके पास खाने तक का समय न था | दिन रात बस मेहनत करता, एक ही अरमान लिए कि उसकी फसल इस बार अच्छी हो और वो पैसे कमाकर धीरे धीरे सरपंच का सारा उधार चुका दे |

उसकी मेहनत रंग लायी | इस बार उसकी फसल इतनी घनी और हरी भरी हुई, कि उसका मन हर्षित हो गया | उस शाम उसने घर जाकर पहली बार सकून से चाय पी और भर पेट खाना भी खाया |

लगेगी" मधु बोली |

"मुझे नहीं जाननी सच्चाई, आप अभी के अभी इस्तीफ़ा दे दीजिये इससे पहले कि कोई और समस्या खड़ी हो" |

इतने में उधर सारे विद्यार्थी एकत्र हो गए | पूनम ने उन सबको मधु के ख़िलाफ़ भड़का दिया | "ये मैडम तुम सबको भी फेल कर देगी एक दिन"|

मधु ने प्रिंसिपल को बहुत मिन्नतें की, 'ये अन्याय है सर, मेरी ये नौकरी मेरा एक ही सहारा है आजीविका का, ये लड़की झूठ बोल रही है' |

"देखिये अभी आप ऐसा कीजिये, दो महीने की छुट्टी भर दीजिये, तब तक मामला ठंडा हो जाएगा, और मैं आपको वापिस बुला लूंगा "

" पक्का सर?"

"जल्दी कीजिये, देखिये बच्चे कैसे हंगामा कर रहे हैं बाहर"

मधु ने प्रिंसिपल के भरोसे घबराहट में छुट्टी भर दी और चली गयी | दो महीने बाद जब उसने प्रिंसिपल को आकर पूछा तो वह मुकर गया अपनी बात से और मधु को पता लगा कि उसके स्थान पर उसने अपने किसी जानकार को नौकरी दे दी | यह सब उसकी खेली साज़िश थी |

मधु का सारा भविष्य खराब हो गया | कोर्ट कचहरियों के चक्कर वो काट नहीं सकती थी, पहले ही उसके घर के हालात ऐसे थे | बेबस होकर वो दो साल घर बैठी रही बिना नौकरी के| इतनी बड़ी कुर्सी पर बैठकर, इतने पढ़े लिखे लोग ऐसे अन्याय करते हैं, तभी हमारा देश विकसित नहीं कर पाता |

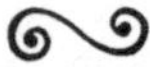

23

अटल सिद्धान्त

आशा के पति का अकस्मात निधन हो गया था | अपने बच्चों का पालन करने हेतु, उसको कोई काम ढूँढना जरूरी था | वह पढ़ी लिखी नारी थी, उसने बी. एड की डिग्री हासिल कर रखी थी | आशा ने जगह जगह अपना इंटरव्यू दिया, पर उसे कहीं नौकरी न मिली | आख़िर में उसका प्रयास सफल रहा और अंततः आशा को एक स्कूल में अध्यापिका के पद पर नौकरी मिल गयी | वेतन थोड़ा कम था, परन्तु अभी उसके जीवन की स्थिति ऐसी थी कि उसको जो भी मिल रहा था, उसे स्वीकार था |

आशा एक अति परिश्रमी और सिद्धांतों वाली अबला थी, जो अपना कार्य पूरी निष्ठा से करती थी | थोड़े ही समय में आशा की काबिलियत पूरे विद्यालय में नज़र आने लगी | उसके पढ़ाये शिक्षार्थी अच्छे परिणाम लेकर आने लगे |

आशा को तीन महीने हो चुके थे, उसी स्कूल में |

एक दिन उसे स्कूल के मुख्याध्यापक ने अपने कक्ष में बुलाया | आशा थोड़ी हैरान थी, पता नहीं सर ने क्यों अचानक से बुलाया है आज मुझे

डरते डरते वो चली गयी |

"सर, मे आई कम इन?"

"आइये, आशा जी, बैठिये, और कैसा चल रहा है आपका कार्य?"

कठपुतली बनकर रह गयी वो, बाहर भी और घर में भी | उन पैसों में से वो अपने भाइयों में लिए भी बचा न सकती थी, सभी उसकी चाची छीन लेती थी |

आस पास बच्चों को स्कूल जाता देख, अच्छे कपड़े देख, माता पिता का हाथ पकड़े देख उसके मन में पीड़ा उठती थी बहुत, "काश आप हमारे पास होते माँ बाबूजी, कौन पूरे करेगा अब मेरे सपने"|

संध्या को रोते देख उसके चाचा से रहा न गया, एक दिन उन्होंने बहुत सोचा कि किस तरह वे संध्या की मदद करें | उन्होंने तय कर लिया कि अब पीछे नहीं हटेंगे |

वे संध्या के पास गए और उसको गोदी में बिठाया और प्यार से सराहा तथा उसके आँसू पोंछे| "पढ़ाई करेगी बेटा?"

"जी, चाचू, मुझे तो बड़ा शौक है पढ़ने लिखने का"

"चल ठीक है, रो मत, मैं पढ़ाऊँगा तुझे"

"पर देख, तेरी चाची को न पता चलने पाए, तुझे पता ही है उसके स्वभाव का", चाचा बोले

"जी, चाचू, मैं ध्यान रखूँगी"

"ठीक है, ऐसा करेंगे, जब तू सर्कस पर जाती है, वहीं से मैं तुझे लेने आ जाया करूँगा और तुझे पढ़ा दिया करूँगा"

"अब ख़ुश ? चल रोना बंद कर अब"

अगले दिन संध्या के चाचा ने उसके लिए किताबें और पढ़ाई का पर्याप्त सामान ख़रीद लिया और संध्या को पढ़ाना शुरू कर दिया | संध्या का दिमाग़ तेज़ था, उसने जल्दी ही पढ़ाई में पकड़ हासिल कर ली | देखते ही देखते संध्या की दसवीं की परीक्षा भी उत्तीर्ण हो गयी और उसकी चाची को ख़बर तक न हुई |

संध्या के चाचा को संध्या पर गर्व था और वे उसे आगे भी पढ़ता देखना चाहते थे |

संध्या ने उनके सहयोग और आशीर्वाद से बी एड की डिग्री हासिल कर ली | आज संध्या एक पढ़ी लिखी कन्या बन गयी | पर चाची की नज़रों में वो आज भी वही घरेलू काम काजी संध्या थी |

एक दिन उनके घर पर कोई समाज सेवक मण्डल आया और संध्या के चाचा के बारे पूछने लगे | वे किसी काम से बाहर गए थे | तो उन्होंने उसकी चाची से ही बात की | जाते जाते उन्होंने कुछ कागज़ निकाले, जिनपर उसको दस्तख़त करने को कहा | संध्या की चाची बिना उनको पढ़े उनपर दस्तख़त करने लगी, तो संध्या ने एक दम बोला," "रुकिए चाची, ऐसे बिना पढ़े दस्तख़त नहीं करने चाहियें, लाइए मुझे दीजिये मैं एक बार पढ़ लेती हूँ, इनमें क्या लिखा है"|

"तू? तू क्या पढ़ेगी ? तेरे को क्या पढ़ना आता ?"

"अरे भाई साहब, इसकी बातों में न आइये, लाइए कहाँ करने हैं दस्तख़त, बताइये"

मण्डली वालों के माथे पर पसीना आ गया, मानो उनकी कोई पोल खुल जाएगी |

संध्या को चाची का स्वभाव पता था, पर वह ग़लत थोड़े होने देती कुछ, उसने उनके हाथ से कागज़ छीन लिए और पढ़ने लगी |

"ये क्या लिखा है इनमें "हर माह, मैं अपनी मर्जी से 50,000 रूपये दान में देता/ देती हूँ"

क्या 50,000 ? चाची बोली |

"पागल तो नहीं हो गयी तू, ध्यान से पढ़ा भी है, पढ़ना लिखना आता नहीं, बात कर रही है?"

चाची मैं सच कह रही हूँ, रुकिए आपको यकीन नहीं मुझपर, मैं पड़ोस से बंटी भैया को बुलाकर लाती हूँ, वो पढ़कर बताएँगे आपको |

संध्या तुरंत गयी और उनको बुलाकर लाई |

"आ जाएँगे काम समाप्त होते ही, तू चिंता न कर", भाभी बोली |

तीन-चार दिन बीत गए, प्रिया को सब टालते रहे किसी न किसी बहाने से |

आख़िर रक्षाबन्धन का दिन आ गया | प्रिया ने ज़िद्द पकड़ ली कि आज तो वो अपने भैया से मिलकर रहेगी, चाहे उसे उनके ऑफिस ही क्यों न जाना पड़े |

"मेरे को जाना है भैया के पास अभी, आज राखी है, इसीलिए तो मैं इतनी दूर से आई हूँ, इतने बरसों बाद, और भैया को राखी बाँधे बिना मेरा मन नहीं मानेगा" |

"पर प्रिया सुन,," भाभी बोली |

"कोई पर वर कुछ नहीं भाभी, इतने दिन हो गए मुझे आए, मेरी बात तक नहीं हुई भैया से, आप मुझे अभी लेकर चलिए उनके पास, नहीं तो."....

"अच्छा ठीक है, चल, रुक मैं ड्राइवर को बुला लूँ गाड़ी लेकर आ जाएगा" |

प्रिया हाथ में राखी की थाली लिए मुस्कुराते हुए चल पड़ती है अपनी भाभी के साथ |

गाड़ी आई और दोनों बैठ गए | प्रिया सारे रास्ते बोली जा रही थी और उसकी भाभी ख़ामोश सी बैठी रही |

"भाभी और कितनी दूर है भैया का ऑफिस ?"

"बस आ गया "

जैसे ही गाड़ी रुकी तो सामने एक अस्पताल की बिल्डिंग थी | प्रिया देखकर दंग रह गयी "अरे भाभी, ये कहाँ ले आई आप ? ये कोई ऑफिस तो नहीं लग रहा"

"तू चल बताती हूँ", भाभी बोली |

प्रिया मन ही मन घबरा रही थी, आख़िर क्या बात है |

अंतत: प्रिया की भाभी को उसे सब सच बताना पड़ा |

सुनकर प्रिया की आँखों से आँसूं नहीं निकले, बल्कि वो पत्थर दिल सी ज़मीन पर गिर पड़ी |

"भाभी ये सब कैसे हुआ, और मुझे किसी ने बताया तक नहीं"

"बस क्या बताते तुझे, सोचा तू इतनी दूर परेशान ही होगी"

प्रिया तुरंत उठी और भाभी को बोला कि उसे अभी मिलना है भैया से |

भाभी ने कहा कि उनसे कोई नहीं मिल सकता, डॉक्टर मना करते हैं |

"ऐसे कैसे मना करेंगे वो मुझे, आज राखी है, और एक बहन को नहीं रोक सकते वो अपने भाई से मिलने को" प्रिया घबराती हुई बोली और चल पड़ी रमेश के कमरे की ओर |

बाहर नर्स ने रोक दिया | जब प्रिया ने हठ न छोड़ी, तो नर्स ने डॉक्टर को बुलाया |

"आप नहीं मिल सकती उनसे, उनकी हालत नाज़ुक है अभी, न होश है उनको" डॉक्टर बोला |

    "आपको पता है आज कौन सा दिन है डॉक्टर ? राखी का, आज आप एक भाई बहन को नहीं रोक सकते मिलने से" प्रिया बोली |

लेकिन,,,डॉक्टर बोला |

"देखिये डॉक्टर साहब, आपको भी मालूम होगा, ये राखी का धागा भले नाज़ुक सा हो, पर इसका जोड़ कितना मज़बूत होता है, और आप भी कहते हैं कि कई बार दवा से ज्यादा दुआ काम आती है, हो सकता है इस रेशम के धागे से ही कोई करिश्मा हो जाए" | प्रिया बोली |

29

एक शिक्षिका का विश्वास

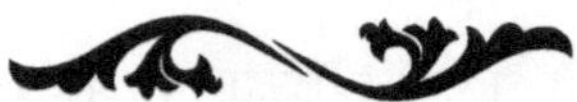

रेनू एक बड़ी होनहार लड़की थी और पढ़ाई लिखाई में बचपन से ही अव्वल रही | उसने अपनी मेहनत और लगन से डॉक्टरी की डिग्री हासिल की | अब वह और आगे पढ़ना चाहती थी | उसने परीक्षा पास की और उच्च स्तरीय शिक्षा के लिए दाख़िला लिया | जिस कॉलेज में रेनू का दाख़िला हुआ, वो माना हुआ शिक्षा सदन था | और वहाँ पढ़ाने वाले सभी शिक्षक भी बेहद क़ाबिल और योग्यवान थे | रेनू बहुत ख़ुश थी कि उसको ऐसी उच्च जगह पर पढ़ने का अवसर मिलेगा |

दाख़िले के बाद कॉलेज जाने का समय आ गया | रेनू अपना बैग लेकर कॉलेज के लिए चल दी | जाते ही अपने सहपाठियों से मिली और सभी शिक्षकों से | रेनू के चार शिक्षक थे | और हर शिक्षार्थी को एक शिक्षक के प्रशिक्षण में अपना कोर्स करना होता था | और उनके कोर्स की एक मुख्याध्यक्षा थी | वो थोड़ी अजीब किस्म की शिक्षिका थी | उसका व्यवहार रेनू के प्रति पहले दिन से ही ठीक नहीं था | बिना वज़ह से वो रेनू को डाँट लगाती रहती थी, सजा देती रहती थी |

रेनू अपनी मेहनत से सारे काम ख़ुद करती थी, जबकि उसके सहपाठी किसी और की मदद से, छल कपट करके अपना कार्य करवा लेते थे | रेनू अपने सेमिनार देती, और उसकी मुख्याध्यक्षा उसको डाँट फ़टकार कर उसका सेमिनार रद्द कर देती थी | रेनू को जान बूझ कर हताश करती थी वो | और बार बार धमकी देती थी, कि डिग्री हासिल करके दिखा ज़रा तू, देखती हूँ कैसे करेगी हासिल |

रेनू की पढ़ाई तीन साल की थी | उसकी मुख्याध्यक्षा के अत्याचार से तंग आकर वो कई बार पढ़ाई छोड़ने का सोच लेती थी, फिर सोचती कि माँ बाप ने इतना ख़र्चा किया उसकी पढ़ाई पर, उसको व्यर्थ कैसे जाने दे | जैसे कैसे वो वक़्त काटती रही | पर भीतर ही भीतर वो डिप्रेशन का शिकार हो रही थी |

रेनू की अपनी शिक्षिका, उसकी मुख्याध्यक्षा की चचेरी बहन थी, पर दोनों में ज़मीन आसमान का अंतर् था | वो हमेशा रेनू को प्रोत्साहित करती थी | जब रेनू का सेमिनार रद्द होता, तो उसकी शिक्षिका पीछे से तालियाँ बजाती और उसको शाबाशी देती | वो रेनू को जो कुछ भी काम दिया करती, रेनू उसे बड़ी शिद्द्त से पूरा करती | उसकी शिक्षिका थोड़ी कड़ी ज़रूर थी, पर सिर्फ़ शिक्षार्थियों के भले के लिए, अंदर से उनका हृदय माँ की तरह कोमल था |

एक दिन रेनू तंग आकर अपनी शिक्षिका के पास गयी "मैम, मैं और आगे अपनी पढ़ाई नहीं कर पाऊँगी, मुख्याध्यक्षा के अत्याचार सहने को क्षमता और नहीं रही मुझमें", रेनू की आँखों से आंसूं आ गए |

उसे उस हाल में देख, रेनू की शिक्षिका चिंतित हो गयी | उनको रेनू की योग्यता पर पूर्ण विश्वास था | उन्होंने रेनू को अपने पास बिठाया और समझाया "बेटा, तुम्हें मालूम है न कोई भी हुनर हासिल करने के लिए इंसान को बहुत कठिनाइयों का सामना करना पड़ता है, ज़िंदगी का यह सफ़र इतना आसान नहीं जितना लगता है | और तुम ये भूल गयी कि तुम्हारे माँ पापा ने तुम्हारे ख़ातिर कितना संघर्ष किया, उनकी एक एक पूँजी मेहनत से कमाई हुई है, जो उन्होंने तुम्हारे सपने पूरे करने में लगा दी, क्या उसे यूँ ही व्यर्थ जाने दोगी तुम?"

"पर मैम, वो मैम तो मुझे डफर बुलाती हैं, हमेंशा यही कहती हैं कि तू कभी डिग्री हासिल नहीं कर सकेगी, जबकि मैं अपना हर काम समय पर करती हूँ और अपनी मेहनत से"

"अरे बेटा, किसी के कहने से क्या कोई वही बन जाता है, जो उसकी सोच हो, हमें खुद पता होना चाहिए कि हम में क्या काबिलियत है, क्या योग्यता है, और देख, हीरे की परख एक जोहरी को ही हो सकती है, जितना मैं तुम्हें जानती हूँ, देखना एक

बोलना, कर ही देगा काम | पर बात बिगड़ती जा रही थी | इस बार तो हद हो गयी, पूरे एक महीने उसने काम रोके रखा |

एक दिन उसके कुछ मज़दूर मधु के पास आए और बोलने लगे "आंटी आप हमारे ठेकेदार को पैसे क्यों नहीं देते समय पर, वो हमारी बग़ार नहीं देता, जब पूछो तो कहता आपने पैसे नहीं दिए" |

"क्या, पैसे नहीं दिए ? मैंने तो हमेशा एडवांस पैसे दिए उसको, ऐसे कैसे बोल सकता है वो, मेरी बेटी खुद उसको पैसे देती आई है हर बार" |

मज़दूर हैरान हो गए ये सुनकर |

मधु को लगने लगा कि भूषण कुछ तो गड़बड़ कर रहा है |

उसने अपने बेटे से बात की | बेटे को ज़रूरी काम के कारण छुट्टी नहीं मिल पा रही थी | उसने बोला माँ पड़ोस में दो चार जनों से बात करके देखो | पर किसी पड़ोसी ने कोई पहल न की | फिर उसके बेटे ने फोन पर बात की भूषण के साथ | उसने ऐसे बात की जैसे कुछ हुआ ही न हो| फिर मधु के बेटे ने उससे कहा कि वो आकर मिलेगा अगले इतवार |

जैसे ही राकेश (मधु का बेटा) आया, उसने पहले भूषण के मजदूरों से बात की | मधु ने उनको कहा कि हमने तो तुम्हें कितना सामान भी दिया था, अगर तुम्हें पता हो | इसके बेटे को बाईक भी दे दी, वो भी बिना पैसे के | एक मज़दूर बोला "सामान तो उसने हमसे उसी दिन ले लिया था और बेच भी दिया कबका।हमें धमकाया कि अगर सामान न दिया तो उनको काम से निकाल देगा, हमारे पास कोई सामान नहीं अब | और वो बाईक तो उसने कबकी बेच दी किसी को, आपको नहीं पता ?"

"क्या, बेच दी ? अभी तो उसके कागज़ भी नहीं बदले, वो आर-सी तो अभी भी मेरे नाम है" राकेश बोला |

सबको इतना आश्चर्य हुआ ये सब जानकर |

राकेश ने भूषण को बुलाया और सारी बात पूछी | भूषण साफ़ मुकर गया | पर इतना सब उसके मज़दूर झूठ थोड़े बोलेंगे | जब भूषण नहीं माना, तो राकेश ने अपने एक दोस्त से बात की और उसको सब सच बताया | वो पुलिस इंस्पेक्टर था | उसने राकेश को भूषण के ख़िलाफ़ एक कंप्लेंट दर्ज करने को कहा |

उसके आधार पर भूषण के ख़िलाफ़ कार्यवाही शुरू की गयी | जिसमें भूषण के एक एक गुनाह का पर्दा फाश होने लगा | भूषण ने मधु से पैसे लेकर मजदूरों को दिए ही नहीं और अपने बैंक के खाते में जमा करता रहा वो | उसने मकान के काम में जो भी सामान लगाया, सब डुप्लीकेट, और मधु से ज्यादा पैसे लिए | जो बाईक वो मुफ़्त में अपने बेटे के लिए ले गया था, वो उसने आगे 30,000 रूपये में बेच दी | और तो और मज़दूरों को दिया सामान भी कुछ अपने घर ले गया और कुछ बेच दिया |

सब सच सामने आने के बाद भूषण को अपना गुनाह मानना ही पड़ा | पुलिस ने उसके ख़िलाफ़ केस दर्ज किया और उसको गिरफ़्तार कर लिया |

मधु को ये सब देखकर इतना दुःख हुआ कि अपने बेटे समान होते हुए भी भूषण ने उसको इतना धोख़ा दिया | काव्या ने कहा "मैंने आपको अपने सगे भाई से भी ज्यादा इज़्ज़त दी, फिर भी आपने हमारा भरोसा तोड़ा, न हमने किसी चीज़ की कमी रखी, न माँ ने आपको कभी पैसे के लिए मना किया, आपके मज़दूरों को इतना खिलाया पिलाया, तांकि बाहर का खाकर वे बीमार न हो जाएँ" |

फिर भी मधु और उसके परिवार ने पुलिस से कहकर भूषण के खिलाफ शिकायत वापिस ले ली और उसे छोड़ने को बोल दिया |

भूषण को लेकिन किसी बात का कोई अफ़सोस नहीं था, उसने अपने मुँह से एक बार भी माफ़ी नहीं माँगी |

मधु का बहुत नुकसान हुआ | भूषण ने जो भी दीवारें खड़ी की थी, वो सब ढहने लगी, क्यूँकि उसने सब माल ख़राब लगाया था |

ACKNOWLEDGEMENT

INNSÆI International Lit Fest 22 was organized at SHREE MALLIKARJUN and Chetan Manju Desai College, Canacona, Goa, India on 18th and 19[th]August, 2022. It was INNSÆI Journal that took initiative to organize this international event and announced the book for publication. All the associates of INNSÆI Journal Mr Orbindu Ganga, Dr Sanjeev Kumari Paul, Ms Aditi Barve, Dr Janatha Ramanathan as well as Mr Vedant Teli, Ms. Arya Desai, Ms Simran Ghashi have contributed to the success. Without SHREE MALLIKARJUN and Chetan Manju Desai College, Canacona, Goa, India, it was not possible to visualize the event in reality. The Chairman, Shri. Chetan Manju Desai, Prin. Dr. Manoj Kamat, Dr Purnanand Chari, Dr Rupa Chari as well as their teaching and non-teaching staff have lion's share in making the event a grand success. This book is the eternal memory of the event.

Dr Kalpana Gangatirkar, as an Executive Editor of the book, has added her scholarly remarks on the contributions of poetry from all over India. She has worked painstakingly for the completion of the book. Ms Aditi Barve has minutely taken care of every aspect in the process of publication. It must be noted that Dr Basudeb Paul, West Bengal, contributed his poem as the first submission after release of the Call.

Further, we are thankful to our fellow poets, all our readers, admirers, and all the members of our family and friends. Especially our virtual friends, though we don't know some in person, however they have been very positive and encouraging with their kind, inspiring and loving words. We would like to thank all our contributors for making this book

anthology successful. So, we express our sincere gratitude to all of them for giving their valuable time for it. Last but not the least, we thank the publication team and the Notion Press, for their genuine support, we could accomplish well. We know our words are not enough; however, we thank you all again for making our dream comes true for this anthology. The contribution of Ms. Sweta Kumari is significant in bringing the book in the hands of the readers.
Heartfelt gratitude to all…!!!

Dr Tejaswini Patil Dange
Chief Editor

Dr Kalpana Gangatirkar
Executive Editor

The trenches gave off the stinking flesh
Lacerated in bullets, bayonets, shells, & bombs!

~ **Basudev Paul**

Where alliance knows only to confer and its formless notion silently implies.

~ **Indrani Chatterjee**

17

Meenakshi Goswami

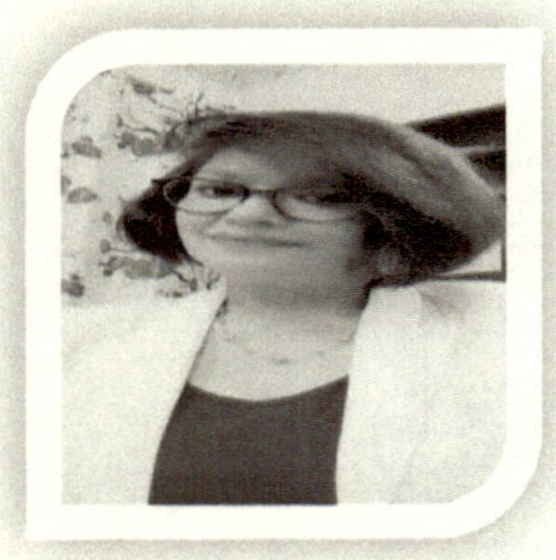

Meenakshi Goswami is the Principal of CNS HS School, Sonitpur Assam and an inhabitant of Tezpur, Assam, India. She has 2 Books of Poems to her credit and also poems are published in many Anthologies. Her debut book *The Sensuous Zephyr* was launched in 2014 in Melbourne Australia where she had attended a Poetry Meet and her Second book *Waltzing Words* is published by the renowned Publisher Authors Press Delhi this 2021 in the month of September. She is a recipient of State Award for Teachers on 5th September 2018 from Govt of Assam and Republic Day Award in 2013 and 2019 for her dedicated service to human resources, Art and Culture. She is also the recipient of Oil Shikshya Ratna Puraskar 2016 in recognition of all round excellence as an educationist. She has attended many multilingual international poetry festivals in India and abroad

Sanguinity

Awoke at aurora by the excruciating sounds of the crackers,
I mizzled for a stroll...

Amid the dissonance I voyaged the cliffs and ridges,
Cruised the riverine,
Applauding the prunes hanging from the twigs and boughs
Apricots and raspberries were glowing in their tender greens
...

Aren't the hills chaste? How weirdly!
Magnificently beautiful that dewy morn
When the crackers were dispensing the anxiety of the hikers
I was but poised
Vanquishing all vagueness,
The breeze at the dawn had the secrets to tell me
I had to look upon it as the quintessence of life,
Nobody can go back and start a new beginning,
Isn't it a serious thing just to be alive?
On this fresh morning- in this broken world -
I arise, start afresh
And keep on strolling flamboyantly...

~ Meenakshi Goswami

From the borders of the poorer to richer countries
So often caught and kept in cubicles
Presented in courts where justice is a game
And the tyranny of money rules
In a world where life and hope
Are fighting a case for asylum
In so many corners, peace is hostage to love!
Held without a word, without a spelt out ransom
Where bullet makers pull up before parliaments
In BMWs and quietly walk in
Peace is hostage to faith and belief!

And on that lovely sunny morning
When instead of holding my face in the palm
Of your hands, you screamed love
And screeched the claim to care
And sent a woman to share my heartbreak
You betrayed the terms of both
Love and peace! And my dear
You won't even pay penalty!

The laws of the land and of the water
Will let you go free! But I won't!
Peace is hostage to dignity!
For every woman on this earth!
And may there be revolutions!
May thunder roar and lightening smile
For all to see and hear!
This world needs to loose all its fear!
Peace is hostage to love!

~ Pankhuri Sinha

33

Dr Shalini Yadav

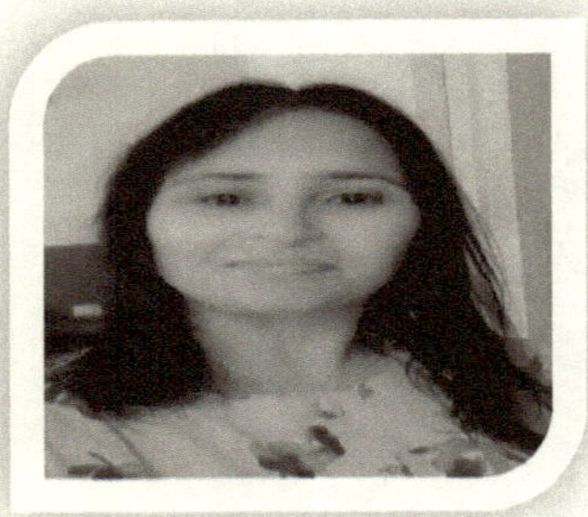

Dr Shalini Yadav is a professor of English and poet from India. She has edited and authored 11 books including three poetry books in English named*Floating Haiku* (2015), *Kinship With You: A Collection of Poems* (2014), *Till the End of Her Subsistence: An Anthology of Poems* (2013), and one in Hindi entitled *Kshitiz Ke Us Paar* (2016). She has recently edited a collection of poetry *Across the Seas* (2022).

Humanity And Peace

Dust and rages take us nowhere,
We all wish to live United here.

A sonless mother with dried tears;
Or a woman trying to save her respect, she wears;
After listening a cry from a heart of a child;
How can we be so barbaric and wild?

All and sundry have the same blood,
Then why to fill the earth with corpses' flood?

Be the ambassador of peace and harmony
Feeding the starving souls a spoon of affection's honey.

It's not so difficult achieving the state of bliss
We just need to discard the demon's kiss.
Embracing and enlivening sensibility,
Can be reroute to positivity and sensitivity.

Battles and Mayhems be the pointless
When we stand together with kindness.

Respect and empathy are humane essence,
Where poetry adds more in the fragrance.

~ Dr Shalini Yadav

All the humbug lovers of the world will be in extreme anxiety.
Give that lover once the rod of an empire-
It's a promise that in millions of years of History, that lover will bury shameless corpse entire.
Let the world save those deprived lovers;
Let them overcome their pain and humiliation, and harmony recovers.

~ Paramita Adhikari

Dr. Sunanda Shelake

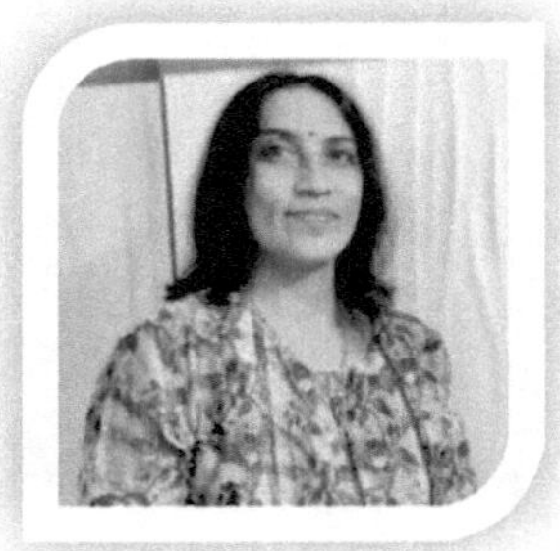

Dr. Sunanda Shelake is a poet from Jaysingpur, Kolhapur, Maharashtra, INDIADr. Sunanda S. Shelake is an Asst. Professor, Research Guide and Head, Department of English. She has been honoured with five Meritorious Teacher Awards. She has 22 Research Papers to her credit. Her other writings including 08 Creative and Critical books has been published. She has also attended several programs of Poetry Reading and Interviews on AIR Sangli. Besides, she has received 38 Awards for creative writing.

At Such Every Time

Whenever I try to grapple with
Every moment of creation
In my eyes there stands
The evergreen tree of love
With new folliage
And underneath my feet
Lies the sleeping silver of moonlight!
However,
My words are unable to
Embrace them with their velvet wings
Comes between
My womanhood!
The anguish of womanhood
Throbs at every threshold
Stumble at the footier of house
At such a time
I think of of bandaging them with the balm of words
However,
Comes between
My tolerant Indian culture!
At such every time
Comes the thought
Needlessly,
Savitri taught me to
READ, WRITE and THINK!
Otherwise,
There would not be
The uneasiness
Underneath the bottom of my words
And there would not have arisen

Savita Vardhaman Patil

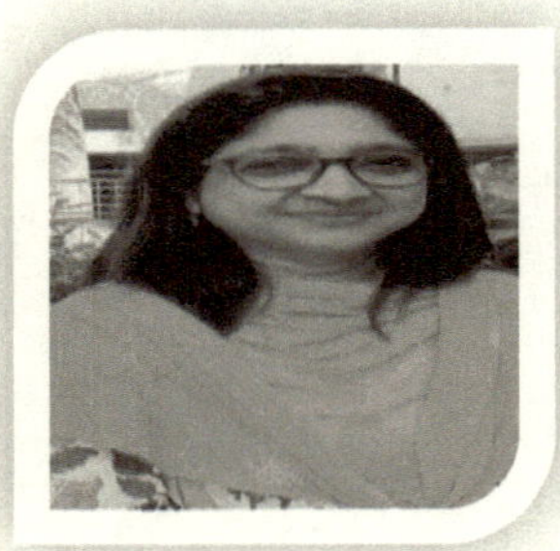

Savita Vardhaman Patil works as a head of English Department in Dr Babasaheb Ambedkar College, Aundh Pune. She has presented many research papers in International, National conferences. Her poems have been published in an International anthology entitled "Feel with You" and in other leading magazines. She is a creative writer and published her short story in volume II entitled "Voices From The Society."

Peace and Humanity

Peace and humanity
are the pillars of human.
Both words are interlinked
and complementary to each other.

Peace and humanity
are found in nature
and in Saints' literature.
But, do we ever get it in human?

Peace and Humanity
are velvet words and
tool of show-off.

The globe has its fate
Of hostile and violent mentality.
Therefore, each one should adopt
Peace and Humanity.

Let the nerves of Peace and humanity
Flow in each personality.

~ Savita Vardhaman Patil

Delightful Destination

The silence,
Between the two tides
Breaking on the shore,
Reverberates the calls of the ocean.

The pause,
Between the rustling leaves
In the forest,
Ascertains the breathing of the tree.

The hiatus
In the cooing of the cuckoo
From the nest
Intuits the soaring of the small wings in future.

They take us
To the delightful destination
With the certitude of the peaceful sleep
In the lap of Nature.

The Bullet

They put a bullet in her head
In front of thousands of like-minded and
The aerial eyes to reach all corners.

The bullet pierced through her brain
Which roused in
 her
An urge to peep out of the thin black linen,
A desire to cross that boundary called threshold
Which was closed to the sky
Her only escape from life.

That impatient organ in her head
Ordered her tongue and vocal chords
To raise her voice against the injustice.

It enhanced her courage
To dive into the books;
To sit in the chairs meant for them;
And proved herself to be equal.

They attacked the very part
Which tempted
Eve to eat the Fruit;
Sojourner to move this Earth upside down;
Elaine or Betty to unfold their Plans;
Savitri to light the lamp of knowledge;
And the Mother to unfurl her compassion to all humanity.

soothed them and erased their fears.

The happy soul with beaming face
taught me humanity is peace and grace.

~ Dr Kalpana Girish Gangatirkar

81

Dr. Sushmindarjeet Kaur

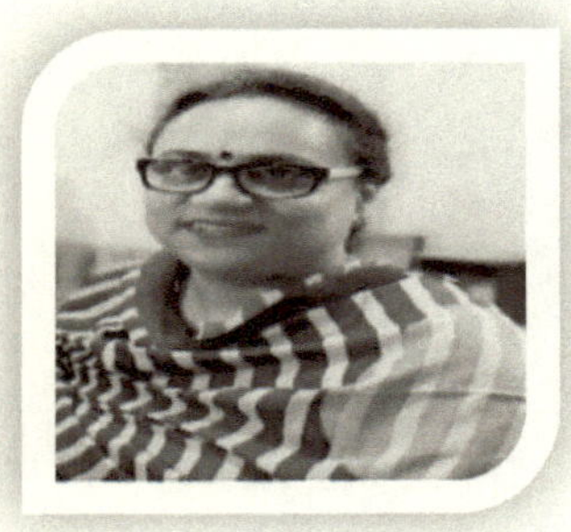

Dr. Sushmindarjeet Kaur is an Associate Professor and Head, PG Department of English at G.G.N. Khalsa College, Ludhiana, Punjab. She has more than 25 years of experience for UG and PG classes. She writes short stories and poetry. She has edited three books. She has translated a book *Sikh Soldiers in Italy during Second World War* which has been published and released in England. She has to her credit more than fifty poems and articles published in various anthologies and journals. Dr Sushmindarjeet Kaur was conferred with Master of Creative Impulse,Philosophique Poetica International Award at World Poetry Conference in 2019. Besides, she has been awarded with the title of Edifying Editor at Poetic Confluence held at Hyderabad in September 2019. She has presented research papers in many International and National seminars and conferences. She is the author of *Voices From Within*, a poetic anthology, besides being the editor of seven books.

Peace

Peace! The articulation sounds perfect and ideal.
Only the word,
And not the state,
As it's not attainable, I suppose.

Yes, how can we realise
We are not aware of?
How can we reflect after discerning?
That, perhaps, is perceptible
 Through our gestures,
Through our words too,
Through our deeds,
Through the act of our performance.

Yes, then perhaps, we become a persona of forgiveness and
clemency,
And a being with compassion
When no urge to demonstrate ourselves,
No craving to ponder upon the trifles,
No motive to live for the sake of *Rasa* of the tongue and ears,
All dwindle and fade away.

That's the state of bliss, harmony, and peace, I suppose.
Attained, though unattainable,
A bit of reticence, quiet,
A bit of introspection,
A bit of forgetting everything,
And
A bit of blessed mind.

~ Dr. Sushmindarjeet Kaur

Table of Contents

(from *Jailhouse Strong: Tactical Shield Training*), the premier tactical athlete Thic Vic (from *Tactical Strongman: The Complete Guide*), and that blue-collar workingman hero Bosco (from *Time Under Tension: Tactical Training*), along with a couple of local prizefighters, a smattering of local gridiron and baseball diamond stars who had made it to the big show, and a few of the incomparable best of the bouncing trade.

It was like we had just stepped into an elite strength guild.

Perhaps the only one who was noticeably absent from this gathering was Chato (from *The Saga of the Tijuana Barbell Club*). The word around town was that he was spending the season in an old adobe just outside of Tulum. Since Chato was far from a social animal, it was difficult to imagine him in this setting, though he most certainly would have had a welcome invitation.

Putting aside our overwhelming feelings of the so-called imposter syndrome, we said our hellos with a type of bashful confidence to those we knew, and Al made the introductions to those we didn't.

After a bit, Al called out to us.

"Hey, fellas, walk with me. I want to show you something."

Walking alongside Al, we heard the soft tinkle of ice against the crystal tumbler holding his single-malt scotch on the rocks.

After a short stroll, we reached a chest-high fence encircling the most magnificent creature of a horse we had ever seen. Its coat was jet-black, save for a splash of white dropping between its eyes and on down its snout.

"This is my pride and joy. This is Mirabello. I bought him from a breeder in Saudi Arabia last year," Al explained. He gazed at the stallion circling the small track with a gait of impossible ease and grace.

"Tell me, when you look at him, what do you see?" he asked inquisitively.

"Strength," we answered in unison.

"Exactly!" Al shouted with such abandon that he threw his arms in the air, spilling drops of scotch on his silk Tommy Bahama shirt.

"Do you know why he looks so strong and moves with a seemingly effortless ease?" Al questioned.

We could have ventured some guesses. But, by this time in our lives, we had been trained in the old school. When you don't know, you listen. So we stayed silent.

A student of some of the most seasoned street scholars from the throwback Italian neighborhoods of the East Coast, Al nodded in approval of our silence and willingness to listen, to learn.

"Fast-twitch muscle recruitment," Al said, answering his own question.

This was a concept with which we had some familiarity. But we remained quiet, with the intent of letting him explain further, so we could learn more. And explain further he did.

Here is what we learned.

What Are Fast-Twitch Muscle Fibers?

Fast-twitch muscle fibers are the largest, most powerful muscular movers in your body. They also have the most potential for growth.

from the rear, and don't forget about the Chippendales stage, where well-shaped butts drive the ladies nuts. Sprints are unsurpassed in building the glutes, hamstrings, thighs, and calves. You can do sit-ups until the cows come home, but your abs will get taxed running at maximum speed (so will your glutes and hammys). But, remember, to get these benefits, you must give 100 percent and run at max speed—this is all while synergistically burning the fat that covers your hidden six-pack and love handles. Properly programmed sprints will simultaneously reduce body fat and inflammation.

10. **Defy aging.** Fast-twitch fibers—use 'em or lose 'em! Far too often, as folks age, they stop moving and train only on machines and sitting down. There's no better way to use fast-twitch muscle fibers than sprinting! Besides, this sprint training can regenerate mitochondria. Why is that significant? Well, as you age, your mitochondria become weaker. All of the not-so-fun aspects of aging – fatigue, fat storage, a decrease in muscle mass, and cognitive decline – are symptoms of impaired mitochondria. So, especially as you age, you want to continue producing new mitochondria to generate as much energy as your cells and organs require. This will give you the ability to live the kind of life you want to live. Basically, sprinting builds power and reaction time so you will be able to react more efficiently to a sucker punch at the high school reunion, make love like an earthquake, jump high, or catch a ball. All abilities that typically fall faster than a drunk on a mountain bike as people age.

This is just the tip of the iceberg and why sprints are the nucleus of this program.

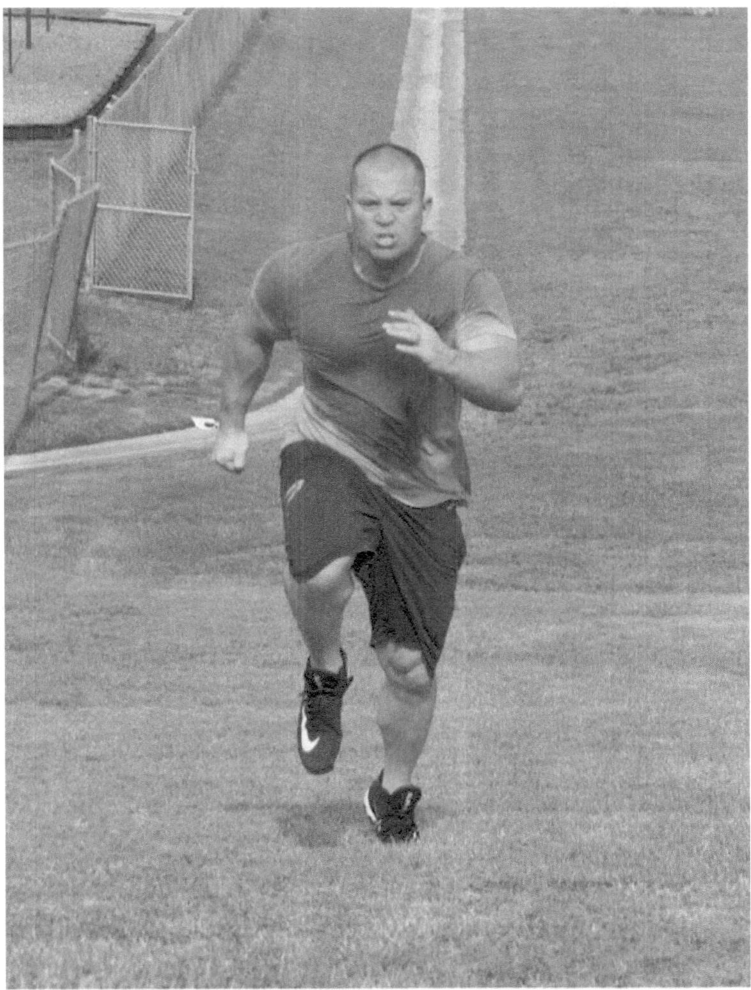

Contrast

Both sprinting and heavy weightlifting rely on fast-twitch muscle fibers to get the job done. Let's take a cursory look at why

BBQ or just giving Coach the confidence to give you the pig-skin every time on 4th and goal—speed strong will get you there.

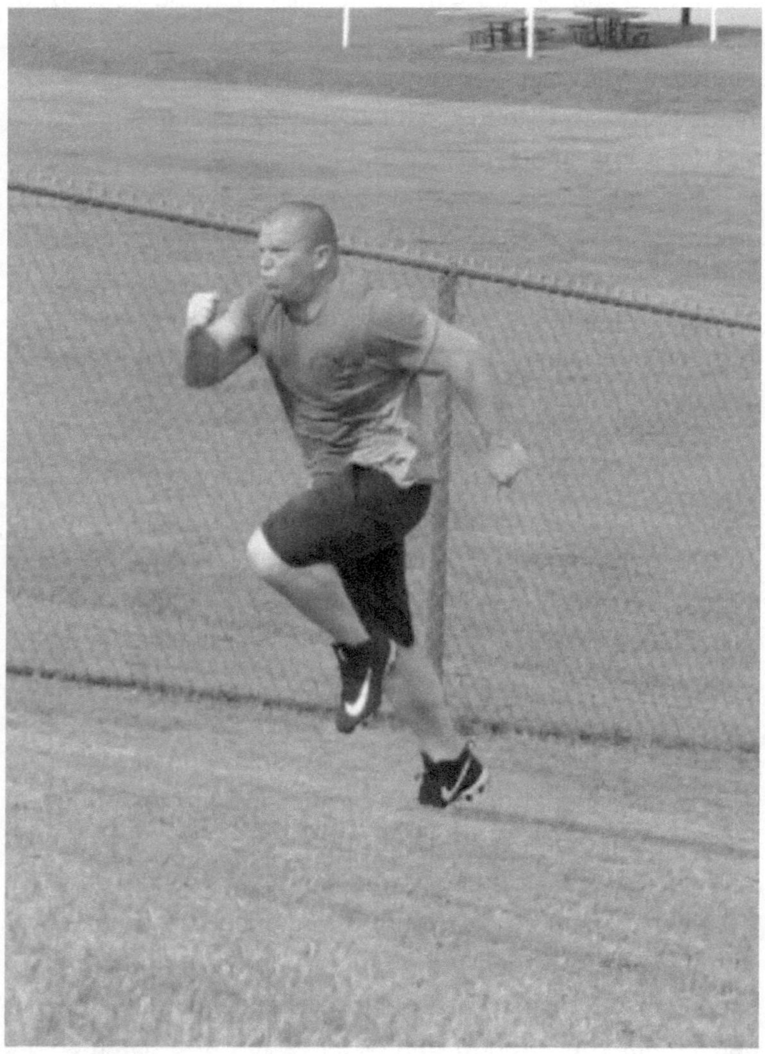

What about you aging athletes?

Left unchecked, Father Time will rob you of movement capacity. You will start every day stiff (the wrong kind of stiff). Speed strong is hard work. But, if you put in the work, you will shrug off flaccidity and begin each morning in a way that would make Coleman tentmakers proud.

In fact, increased movement capacity is one of the real benefits of this particular program for the athlete who has put some miles on his body through hard training, contact sports, and the requirements of a tactical job. By building strength through explosive movement, you will move better and stronger.

Rather than moving with unrestricted liberty, many folks willingly cram their bodies into the confines of a cardio box. As movement capacity declines with age and overuse, taking your place in the hamster wheel on an assembly line of manufactured "workout" machines only exacerbates the problem, like pouring gasoline on a fire. It becomes part of a slow crawl toward decreased functionality and physical ability. You will become the antithesis to staying Gas Station Ready.

Don't shy away from real movement! Break free from the confines of cookie-cutter cardio machines and start moving with Speed Strong!

Sprinting

We covered the benefits of sprinting above. If you are unsure whether you should start sprinting, begin with the Gas Station Ready Hill Sprint program. Go to Joshstrength.com, sign up for the free newsletter, and the free program will be delivered to you. Complete that program before beginning this one.

Speed Strong Program

Day 1
Series 1 (Squat/Sprint)

Set #1	Exercise	Weight	Reps	Rest Interval	Notes
	Squat	80% of 1RM	RPE 7	90-180 sec	
	Sprint	Bodyweight	6 seconds straight		

Set #2	Exercise	Weight	Reps	Rest Interval	Notes
	Squat	90% of 1RM	RPE 9	90-180 sec	
	Sprint	Bodyweight	6 seconds straight		

Set #3	Exercise	Weight	Reps	Rest Interval	Notes
	Squat	75% of 1RM	RPE 9	90-180 sec	
	Sprint	Bodyweight	6 seconds straight		

- Any squat variation is acceptable (high bar, low bar, front squat, belt squat, box squat); use the same variation and depth the entire duration of the program. For all exercises, keep them the same for the entire six weeks of this program.
- For the first three weeks, use the same weight. For the second three weeks, you can add 5 to 10 pounds weekly, regardless of strength levels; if it's too easy, do more reps.
- Sprints are from a dead stop at top speed, immediately after squats. If you do not have somewhere to sprint six seconds or 60 yards (a field or track), you can sprint on a machine for six seconds once top speed is reached or sprint against a band tied to a rack for six seconds, focusing on driving your legs and moving as fast as possible.
- If you are not in condition to sprint at full speed, do sprints up a hill or with a weighted sled with 25 percent of your bodyweight to slow you down. IF IN DOUBT, DO ANOTHER PROGRAM.

Series 2 (Farmer's Walk/Sprint)

Set #1	Exercise	Weight	Reps	Rest Interval	Notes
	Farmer's Walk	75% of deadlift 1RM	50 feet straight	90-180 sec	
	Sprint	Bodyweight	6 seconds straight		

Set #3	Exercise	Weight	Reps	Rest Interval	Notes
	Pendlay Rows	RPE 9	5	75-150 sec	
	Vertical Jumps	Bodyweight	5		

Set #4	Exercise	Weight	Reps	Rest Interval	Notes
	Pendlay Rows	RPE 9	5	75-150 sec	
	Vertical Jumps	Bodyweight	5		

- Pendlay Rows: Dead stop each rep, keep your back flat, and touch the barbell to your upper abdomen.
- For the vertical jumps, swing your arms down and back violently (it's a countermovement vertical jump), and reach up to the sky as you leave the ground.

Day 6 (AKA, Keeping You Chippendales Ready)

Exercise 1

Arnold press: With 15-rep max, go to failure; once failure is reached, do max reps without dropping the dumbbells and continue with regular dumbbell overhead presses. Do this for one set.

Exercise 2

Cable uppercut fly: Start with a 20-rep max; at failure, rest 10 seconds and continue until 100 total reps is reached. Once this is complete in five or fewer sets, you can add weight.

Exercise 3

Overhead rope triceps extensions: Start with a 20-rep max; at failure, rest 10 seconds and continue until 100 total reps is reached. Once this is complete in five or fewer sets, you can add weight.

Exercise 4

Machine biceps curls: Start with a 20-rep max; at failure, rest 10 seconds and continue until 100 total reps is reached. Once this is complete in five or fewer sets, you can add weight.

Exercise 5

Dumbbell lateral raises: Do eight sets of eight reps, with a 20-second break. Keep form very strict.

Day 7 OFF

Final Thoughts

Weakness is a crime, don't be a criminal!

You now have the tools to fight crime, and we look forward to hearing about your results. This program will help you holistically develop a sound mind, body, and spirit!

Contents

attention but my ears were noticing each and every word clearly. I think this was the way we express our deep love. Oh! You can say it Love and hate. It's how our life was crawling without any indication to run. I was always defective and my wife Olivia attacking like the God has given her the right. I chanted so many words in my mind so that I could be the part of her attacking and I think that's the love and hate which always keep us alive but sometimes life takes us to a place from where getting back is really impossible or maybe sometimes very hard to steal and capture the same moment. We don't value the trouble till we face the next bigger trouble in our life.

"We don't have much food for this month; she got frustrated, picked the cloth to clean my messy novels spread everywhere."

I always saw a big revolution in her sparkling eyes but I was not a good master to understand her eyes well like a girl always wanted to and yes, I accepted it, apologized.

"Your daughter Pearl needs new toys every week. What should I do? She continued, settling the handful of novels in my trivial bookshelf. I don't have much patience for your unemployed bearded face."

I had the giant face, unshaved every time because I didn't have much money to shaven it. Huh! I didn't like a beggar. She married to me because I was the most handsome man in her college. We met, greet and then get married. Things were too swift that we never take care of our future. Her angry face was my blush face on those days. She was always the short-tempered girl, a little bit stubborn but a girl with a caring nature and that's made me her husband.

"Why don't you understand that we have a future? She sighed. Our fortune is much worse than anything else. Our children are growing day by day. We need handsome money to teach them in good schools. I don't want my children to grow like you, she screamed aloud at me."

I could see the ocean of tears in her eyes but still on my place holding and crushing every page in my mind to show my mild behaviour. I was also short tempered like her but sometimes to keep the relationship alive we have to do understand each other so that things can be better off than to get worse each and every second.

I was the most ordinary guy in the college except my rare blood group. I had O blood group and that's why my college friends shouted at me by the name **"Rare blood"** every time, and that's how I got popular among the students in my college. Sometimes I felt shame for my jobless position. I couldn't even earn good money for my family. I went to the many offices every day to give a couple of interviews in the hope of getting a good job so that I could bring the soft loaf of bread two times a day for my family, but unfortunately, I was not even capable of that. We lived at the snag in Canada in a small filthy condition wooden house which always encrust with heavy snow each and every second. This wooden house was insanely a deep freezer; you couldn't even sleep without wearing two or three pairs of heavy woollen clothes. I think this place was the coldest place for us nearby, but our poverty-stricken condition was much apathetic than this dangerous winter.

We didn't have so many things in our wooden house except the ancient crockery. We had shattered wooden furniture; a couch whose corners were crushed, some utensils included the ancient crockery which we couldn't sell but only the pieces of emotions of our progeny and a basement full of creepy shit things. If you would see those creepy things in the basement at night, it would look like a didn't know how she came to know the words which were wandering inside our hearts a few minutes ago.

"Darling, have you looked outside? I defend and said cleverly to my wife. Ronan and I were deeply tired not because of the heavy weight of the wooden log but because of the adventurous sight we saw a few seconds ago."

"Not at all! She declared without giving any attention. What's so special about this consistent boring day? I think it's much worse than our past days, she popped again."

I picked sharp knife carefully from her hand and threw it in the plate and that sound was creepy and hold her hand with my cold hand lovingly to take her to the window beside to our main door. I rubbed my soft gloves on the frozen window to remove the fog from the glass. We hardly saw anything from our window because there's nothing special outside except sky lighting and heavy snowfall even our frozen window never allowed us to do so.

"Look at the sky, my angry wife, I whispered in her ear." She twirled her eyes to see outside the window rubbed a few seconds ago, struggling to prevent fog on it."

"Dark giant clouds! She said killingly. Her eyes were still opened in astonishment. I have never seen such drastic moment in my life; she admitted curiously suddenly I picked her beautiful soft hand in excitement to regain the happy moment again."

"Shh! The world is going to end, what about earning so much money in our whole life; I laughed with the thick voice. The fog was still locked in our mouth to get exchanged."

"She cuddled me in excitement. We both were smiling silently. I could see her eyes warm for our love. So, you still angry at me! I asked while rubbing my eyebrows. Ronan and pearl both were looking at her innocently."

"Go and play with your younger brother, I said to Pearl and take care of your little brother Devin as well."

They went while giggling in their manner, showed their white teeth and left to another room.

So, David, what you asked? She smiled, covered her both hands around my neck.

You still angry at me! I asked.

Not at all, she replied silently.

"Look into my eyes and said"

"I really want you to earn more in your life. I want you to grow much stronger than anyone, she suggested, controlling her heavy tears.

"Oh, my sweetheart, I slicked my thumb to wipe her tears. I even want to earn more but I never think about earning money and creating castles. I want my family to be happy. If money makes us happy, then there's no meaning of life. Life is much more than that."

Ridiculously, nature interrupted us, we heard the loud sound of lightning; first, we both frightened and laughed loudly and that was the happy moment I always have. She was laughing confidently and I got the answer to my question. She took my hand and put it on her face. My hands were burning cold but she was still enjoying my frozen hands on her warm face.

You know, David our love is much stronger than this frozen wind. The fire is already lit in our hearts, she whispered in my ears.

"And dear what about the fire in this extinguishing furnace, I said and we laughed again. She twisted my nose and kissed lightly on my lips."

"Okay! Okay! Excellent My love let me fire this furnace, we would have so much time for our lusty love, I said confidently and opened the log of wood in one jerk."

Olivia was seeing my freakish dumb face quietly, controlling her laugh well still I seeing her latent smile. Sometimes I used this trick for Olivia as well when her hands got frozen while working in the office for the whole day."

Pearl kissed my cheeks proudly! And this was the much happier moment than anything else in the world. They went quickly, laughing innocently and I was still managing the ocean of tears in my eyes.

"Olivia! Let's switch on the TV, our bizarre box, have a look at the today news. We don't know from where this Helicopter part fell into our veranda? I think we should call the police. What do you think? Even the weather condition is also getting worse. Today's snowfall is really heavy and horrible."

Yes, sweetheart! She suggested.

"Yeah! And Darling please bring my ponderous fur winter jacket, I really need it. I requested and became stationary on the wooden sofa. My hands were freezing continuously and it was an unbearable situation for me this time."

"Olivia, I asked again but breaking news of the idiot box interrupted us very cleverly."

Canada News

"The weather condition is not much favourable. Temperature is declining even more than our weather predictions. The weather department predictions have already failed. We are reporting from the snag, East Canada. The ice is hard and frozen here. If you look at me, I am wholly covered with the end number of woollen clothes; he yelled, a little bit panicked with the low voice and then adjusted his mike really close to his smoking mouth covered with snow. As you can see, there's only ice and ice everywhere and if we talk about current temperature, its four degree Celsius and still there's no report, no announcement from the weather department. Why is weather department still silent about this sudden decline in temperature? Are we stuck in this area? What should people do to save themselves from this brutal ice wind? You are watching Canada news and I am Andrews Sanz."

"Ugh! Our media always shows each and every news, after snipping so many threads, Olivia yawned. When would they show us true news?"

She was speaking non-stop and I was lost somewhere else.

"David! Olivia said"

"David! She said again, but I halted her in middle of the talk."

"Oh my God! Ronan, I said, inside scared; let's bring the digital temperature machine. Go go go, very fast. It's in the basement of our house; I asked and threw TV remote on the table carelessly."

"David, can you tell me what's going on? She sounded, curious to know what's happening inside my mind."

The partial burning helicopter part in our veranda, then this weather new! Is everything okay? She asked again."

"Olivia listens attentively! Look at the sky, isn't look strange or very strange? We are living or surviving in this dangerous four-degree Celsius temperature. It's very much strange. Everything would freeze. How would we survive? This could be very drastic dear, I said, halted my words forcefully. We have to leave our house right now! I am not getting the positive vibes."

"Dad! Is this the box? Ronan interrupted us, gasped for his breathe and he handed the box to me quickly. I opened the box with my frozen fingers and bring out the laboratory baby's smile of Devin. They were just a few miles away from me but seemed to be very far away from me. How our thinking changes everything in just one blink.

Mom! Dad! The strange girl whispered in my ears. Her voice echoed in my heart, but I was helpless and making an unending spiral of my thoughts which was not allowing me to stop even for any strange girl. I boosted myself but suddenly I saw a big black glossy luxurious car on the one side of road. There was just one car on the road, much glossy than my life. I don't know what had stricken in my mind, but I know I was in hurry to see my family and this forced me to do so. I opened the chain of my jacket, stuffed the girl into it like a kangaroo, and locked it like an airbag. I took the heavy iron rod of the street light, broken few minutes ago and smashed it on the black glossy thick glass of the car, seemed to be strong but not more than me. Few seconds ago, I was seeing my apologized face and after that broke it. The alarm got alarming echoed without my permission. I accumulated all my strength and opened the lavish gate of the car. The girl was started to crying... Hey hey! Please stop crying! I panicked a little bit. *Even I don't know how to stop the crying of a baby girl and how could I know, I was never decided to be a good dad.* I managed to get into the car and punched hard into the lavish odometer, bring out the expected wire, and ignite the engine cleverly. The alarm was continuously frustrating both of us, till I got disconnected the wires. I turned off the GPS quickly and turned the lavish steering to my way. I had never driven such type of luxurious car in my whole life. There were only hard melting ice and frozen dead bodies everywhere on the road. I didn't want to drive over the dead bodies and I know, maybe some of them were alive. My hands were still trembling to drive over them, but my eyes got astonished when I saw at the temperature, it was -2.5 degree Celsius. I was thrilled and tensed to see the extreme low temperature, and somewhere little bit confused. I was driving the car carelessly, partially out of control due to slippery road and sometimes upon the bodies laid on the road everywhere. I was just few steps from my home, but that was looking far away than we had journeyed. I was driving the car, but that was not the end, my heart got terrified when I saw a blizzard of ice coming towards just opposite to our direction. We were going to collide with the tornado. To reduce the attacking velocity, I stopped the car in between the road to face the tornado, making a spiral of snowy wind with heavy icebergs. It was coming toward us like a huge fire. In just microseconds we stuck with it, the car jumped and waved high in the air. The car started the alarm again. The storm jerked us completely from inside. Suddenly the alarm stopped and car fell on the ground, settled on the wheels, made heavy noise. Windows were a little bit cracked and an airbag was swollen automatically and this time it saved us from deep struck with the steering and that's how rich people save them from accidents and sprinkle sand into the eyes of death. In just few seconds we reached and I parked the car randomly in front of the road. My heart sunk and shocked when I saw the broken condition of my wooden house. It was completely destroyed and covered with ice. I yelled high, ran towards the broken remains, trying to remove the ice, getting hard from the wood. My eyes were deep red and I was really angry at myself to left my family alone in this tough situation. I was cursing myself again and again. The injured anonymous girl in the car was still staring at me. How could the God much worse to take away the life of my family? I was still trying to remove the frozen logs of wood destruction, Henry gasped his breath, waiting for some positive feedback from the head Ms Arden."

"So, the gentleman you think, this is Skyfall, she sounded clever and picked the book in her hands. The book was a little bit dusty, ancient and stuffed with rough yellow pages, printed in some old fonts. She opened and checked some pages, tore at the corners and accidentally she found an old bookmark on page number seventy-two."

Page number 72, Skyfall

"We need to save our self from the curse of nature. This is the way how god shows their resentment on us. People think that they are God just by earning few pennies in their pocket and getting some good knowledge, proving themselves a good gentleman, but in reality, the human can never become God. The world is always in the sacred hands of God. Earth is our mother and if we don't take care of it, it would vanish her. Everything has an end. To save ourselves we need to leave because no one can stop nature except the magic of God. Nature has much time to destroy us, but we have only a few seconds to save us."

Everything got silent and she put the book calmly on the table.

"So, how can we save people? She triggered, inside agreed on his opinion and why it after hundred years? And why should we believe you?

"Do you have any option? He said unthinkingly, ignored her former question.

Jay, one of the team members, asks the media team to get ready, she ordered him. We need to inform public as soon as possible, she smiled in clever gesture and Henry accepted her smile.

Few seconds were passed just after they got agreed but I think God had decided something different for us. The spiky ice cone-shaped shattered the window one after the other and directly stitched into the head of Arden with the tremendous speed. I was really astonished what was happening there. The drops of blood fell everywhere on the surface and the cover of the book but it was not the end, the razor pointed ice passed her head entirely and its tail ended by opening her dead mouth. She fell on the surface in microseconds and a line flashed in her mind abruptly, "Nature has much time to destroy us, but we have only a few seconds to save us".

Oh shit! Shit! Henry screamed, wanted to speak more but stunned even everyone got stunned and the end number of spiky cone-shaped ice entered the room one after one. Three men fell on the ground in just one jerk, three were escaped, screaming and trying to save their lives. I grabbed the book swiftly and came out from the weather department room into the main hall. People were felling on the ground due to slippery ice. Blood and spiky cone-shaped swords everyone. The surface was much slippery and I also slipped on it and a spiky cone of ice hit directly on my left leg. I yelled in pain, controlled myself and hide near the entrance gate of the hall. A screaming voice was echoed in the hall. Everyone was trying to escape through the lift, stuffed into it like the dead bodies. After few minutes I managed to crawl towards the lift. The book was still stuck in the left pocket of my pants. People were trying to enter the lift without caring for others, not even for ladies and children.

"Please come out, Henry yelled and tried to control the situation but no one wanted to leave. Please come out! He requested again. They all were frightened, mad and didn't want to listen to anyone. They just wanted to save themselves. No one wanted to leave and this time it

CHAPTER FIVE

Snag, Canada

1 o clock Sunday Afternoon

Sun would not rise in this country for the next one year, Henry declared while checking the book "Skyfall" whose pages had gone wet due to snowfall. The ink of the yellow pages was vanishing and partially visible. Spiky cone-shaped swords were still falling from the sky even much bigger than the before from the last two days.

"What? David astonished, looking at him into the side view mirror of the car. Sun will not rise for one year! Have you gone mad? By the way, who are you? We would drop you at the next safe place. Be ready!"

"So you think there's some safe place ahead. Good job man! Excellent job! He laughed a bit. You will not find any safe place even not in this country right now."

"Whatever! We would drop you at the next, whether safe or not, we don't bother, David declared without any humanity."

"What? Olivia his wife interrupted him in the middle! How can you do this David?" Look at her! Her hand is bleeding and broken. Blood is flowing from her deep cut wound. Are you becoming selfish for yourself, she yelled, offended inside!

"Yeah! I am selfish. I am selfish for my family. I want to save my family. We don't have anything. No food, no shelter, how can you think about helping a stranger, what do you have? What can you give them? We have a car whose diesel is going to empty in few hours, David spluttered, gripped his hand tightly on the lavish steering."

Hey listen, both of you, we can't help you. We have lost our little baby in this blizzard and I don't want to lose my family. "Temperature is favourable and we have to find a safe place to stay with my family at night; he sobbed. And how can you say that sun would not rise? Why we trust you? Obviously, you are a stranger. We can't trust you anymore."

And David stops the car in the middle of the road, full of snow up to 2 feet, only allowing the car to crawl.

"David, you can't do this, Olivia said unconsciously."

"I can help you! Henry insisted me. I can take you out from this blizzard. I know everything about this. Only I can save you from this. Are you getting what I am saying?"

"I can't...... suddenly the Pearl picked my bare hand tightly, with the intention to stop me. Dad, please! I was still seeing the faces of everyone and my mouth was stitched with her love. I didn't want to break her heart. I accepted her decision closed the door."

"Sir! Look outside and see these spiky cone-shaped ice swords, listen to the disturbing voice and tell me, would we really able to save our self? Henry said and pick out the book from his pocket again. Canada is going to end in next two days and you would not be able to do anything except seeing the destruction under your nose. When God wants new beginnings, he takes the help of nature. Do you want to bury under the graveyard of ice? This is not a normal ice fall, this is Skyfall!

"What! What did you say? David got astonished. Before Henry explained further the roof of the car got bulged

"Suddenly Olivia put her right hand on my back silently. David! We have lost our baby and I would not apologise you for this until the end of my life, she said quietly. I want divorce. I can't live with you anymore."

"I nodded my head quietly. I would not even apologise, I cursed to myself."

"Dad! I am thirsty; Pearl picked my hand innocently with the sad face. My throat is paining Dad. I need water."

I looked at Olivia, still, some hope was lost inside me but she showed her back like a stranger as I expected. Pearl didn't ask me for the water again. She saw everything and I think she understands that much. God has given magical power to understand the complicated things well and we grow and lose that power.

"Come with me, I said in belief. The twisted waves of thoughts were still wandering into my mind, teasing me each and every moment and I really don't know why? In just two days I have seen the hell and heaven both."

I took the empty bottle from the dicky.

"You love white, soft snow? I questioned pearl, to enlighten her face. I never want my children to live with the sad face."

Yes, Dad! She replied, showed the smiling face. We were in the car. I took some soft snow and stuffed it directly into the bottle and put it inside my jacket to get it warm so that the ice can melt with my body heat and she would get water to drink. Olivia was not much happy with me and I think this was the last time when I could do something for my family.

Dad, look! Pearl interrupted me in the middle.

I was still lost in my thoughts.

Dad, look?

What?

Look! What have I written?

She had written "Dad with the smiling face" from the fog, waiting to get melted on the glass window.

She always did something to make me happy. We should do anything to make our family happy. How ridiculous the jokes are, we should enjoy. One day we would see back and realised they were good jokes. I kissed her forehead with my cold lips.

"Hope to see more from you dear, I sounded, nodded my head and smiled for few seconds."

"And she smiled innocently."

"Lenore screamed! Come here, all of you come here."

We got scared as we fed up with the problems now and ran towards her.

"Look at this bag! Is it yours? She starred at me. I found this under the seat of the car."

"It's not mine, obviously the car is not mine, so it's not mine, I declared, showing the clever face. Open and Check it! What's inside?"

"Be careful, Henry interrupted in the middle."

Yup and she opened the bag in just one jerk, its sound echoed and still lost in the sky.

"Oh, I think it's not yours Mr David, she targeted me."

"Yeah obviously! Not mine. I replied."

Everyone was stunned. It was full of million dollars filled at every corner systematically.

"Now it's ours! Henry declared unthinkingly."

"How can you say? No, no it's not ours, I insisted."

"But this bag found in this car? We can take it."

"No, we can't. I stole the car just to save us. We can't take this. I am selfish but I am not greedy."

"But this money is for the safety of your family!"

'What safety? You think money can still save us?"

CHAPTER EIGHT

Snag, Canada

11 o clock Sunday Night

Same day

We were still moving into the woods with the scared faces and the empty stomach. Our eyes were waiting for the unexpected magic but it doesn't happen before we believe ourselves. Everything was frozen around us. The chill snowy wind was going deadly. We were seeing the trees but not seeing the greener leaves on it. It was looking like wandering into the dream heaven peacefully but it was not like that to spend whole life there.

"Dad I am hungry, Ronan said tonelessly. He turned his eyes towards me, looking tired, pale and weak. His hairs were felled carelessly on his head. I was worried about all as we have not eaten anything from the last three days."

"Ronan, wait! You are a brave boy, I replied in the negative gesture which I didn't want to show but I was regretting myself for doing an incurable sin for my whole life. When I had time, I never took care of them and now I wanted to but I didn't have anything to do. Olivia's eyes were closed and she was not looking at me. We have to reach the USA and then she would take divorce with me. I was totally confused whether to save my family or to save my relationship.

"Hey listen to David! Henry said, rolling his fingers over the steering."

"Olivia and I nodded, partially ignored him."

"I know the departmental store where we can get a lot of fresh food. We can eat and store it too, Henry said again, slowing the speed of the car and we jumped unintentionally in the air."

"So, you think, that departmental store is still safe, even in this drastic Skyfall, I asked cleverly to Henry."

Maybe it could be safe and I think should be because it's the only departmental store in this area, that can save us from starving, Henry grinned and moved the steering smoothly to the left turn. Spiky cone-shaped ices were rolling and striking with the car tyres, damaging each and every moment.

"Do you have any good news? I said insanely."

"Yes! I have, Henry replied. I think he was making fun of me. We are still alive even after the life taking Skyfall but I don't know about the future and he straightens his eyebrows. There was still the moment of chaos inside the car.

"Hey you all, Henry announced, grabbed steering, shoe on the accelerator properly. Tighten your seatbelts and grabbed the hand of each other tightly. We are going to jump over a fifteen feet mountain of snow."

You must be joking, Olivia ignored.

"No, I am not, Henry replied. We don't have any other option."

We screamed aloud in the air that teased our ears entirely. His hands were trembling over the steering and eyeballs were on the ice mountain. Ronan grabbed the hand of his mother tightly.

"Okay! She agreed. So, we have to make a tent, maybe canvas tent or....... Lenore said."

"We don't have the canvas to make any tent that can bear this temperature. I said, starring at her for an answer."

"But we have the lengthy bonnet, to bend it from the middle and make it like a roof, she replied smartly. Of course, we can do this from the lengthy bonnet. Please give me a tool to do a hole in the deep ice, she asked to me."

"Will it be safe? Olivia asked."

"Not sure, but I think safe than moving in this weather."

"There's a hammer, I said."

"Give me, she said and stuck hard into the ice to make some deep holes."

We were fortunate that ice was hard. A harsh voice echoed in the air. Suddenly hard ice got cracked like partitioned into two pieces. Before she said something, we all jumped to her side abruptly.

Oh shit! This was not the land, this was the frozen river. Run! Run! Olivia screamed. David grabbed the hand of both children. We have to move, Lenore yelled and picked the hand of little strange girl tightly.

We had no chance. Suddenly she kicked the bonnet get it inverted. We all jumped on it and pick the sharp sides tightly; she announced and tightens her hairs to do ski, first time with the bonnet. She pushed the bonnet with her legs and get into it swiftly. We were moving fast and randomly on the ice, sliding like a ride on the melting ice, but didn't know where we were going. Everyone was yelling, controlling each other. The crack partitioned of the river was following us like the angry police. We didn't know what we were doing but we found it safe rather than waiting for the death. The brutal adventure seized us tightly. Before we could think anything, we saw someone who was blinking the lights of a vehicle. It was two circular lights something like he was giving the indication to us to come forward. Lenore understood it well and brings out her leg ahead and rubbed on the snow to change our direction towards the source of light. We were only seeing the lights and snowballs which were beating us harshly. Our skin was frozen and our patience was getting unbearable. We were still falling into the swift speed, impossible to stop, suddenly the slope ended and our speed came to slow down but the blizzard was still following us even more than the greater speed we thought. When we zoom our eyes, it was a source of dark light from a big bully car, looking like an ambulance. We sloped down and close to it, a man with the hat, whose colour was not visible in the dark, but it was looking black due to reflection fall on it. Suddenly he threw the rope high into the air, stuck by the ice balls and swift wind in the air. Lenore jumped high to catch the rope. The Vehicle got started and we were moving into the random directions struggling to get rid of the bullshit blizzard. We were jumping and bumping high into the air due to icebergs. After five minutes of struggle, we fell carelessly on the snow swiftly when the vehicle stopped. Our bodies were frozen totally, waiting for the help. We were only seeing the man, who came out of the car to help us.

"You are still alive, the man in the brown hat replied. Now the colour of his hat and our hope was looking visible. He was the man with a bunch of hairs, round face, with brown eyes, sparkling in the dark night."

"Hey come inside, He said, opened the gate of the ambulance. There was too much cold. Hey, the little girl comes inside, he asked pearl."

The speed was about eighty kilometres per hour. This ambulance can't bear the weight of this blizzard. We have to move swiftly otherwise we all will bury. We are hardly ten kilometres away from the airport, she declared, struggling to see through the broken glass.

Before we reached the hat of the doctor flown away with the wind.

"Hey! What you did, the doctor yelled. It was my lucky hat."

"Hope the hat blew away and you are still safe. I think you are the lucky one who is still safe, she mumbled, turning the hard steering to the right."

"See there's the long run away. The airport must be there, Olivia said, showing the way to Lenore."

She turned the steering to the right smoothly and stopped just in front of the giant iceberg.

"No no it was an airport, no iceberg, okay let's see, she said, much confused inside."

It was looking like a huge iceberg but before it was an airport because somewhere the shiny glass was reflecting light into the sky.

"Where's the airport, the doctor said, while looking out of the window?"

"In front of you, Lenore said, gasping for breathes."

"Is this the airport? The doctor said again. Look at the runway. There's hardly any space to walk on it and we are going to run a plane. I think we have gone mad."

"Look, just before us, a plane arrived here. They must be inside, Lenore guessed. There's also the back side of the runway."

"Okay! Okay, but how will you get inside, Olivia interrupted."

Before we plan anything, Lenore gets into van swiftly.

"Pick your seats tightly, she said."

"What you are going to do? The doctor astonished."

"We will smash this huge iceberg, she declared, pushed the accelerator cleverly and in few seconds, we stuck with the thick ice wall. It was a huge jerk even drastic than any earthquake and we got inside. Suddenly the ice falls on the entry gate again and gate got vanished without any indication to do so. We have already entered into it. It was really like a freezer, big bully freezer to freeze each and every bone of the human.

"Don't say we are locked inside here, the strange woman asked."

"I think we are, huh! Olivia yelled at her herself."

We came out from the van to see what is going outside.

The flight is going to America, will leave in few minutes. Kindly pass about the security system and take your seats, thank you, a voice from the speaker echoed inside the airport.

"Is everything all right? I yelled, still inside the ambulance van."

"Everything is all right! Lenore answered. Men are dead and machines are still alive! Wow!

"Take him out, Lenore said to Olivia."

"Hey look straight out of the window, Dr, Carl said astonishingly. There are some people who can help us."

They were looking like commandoes in black uniforms, shielded with weapons, standing near a plane. We ran towards them swiftly and stopped under the small roof where they were standing.

"Please help us. Two injured persons are with us. Please help us, Olivia said, crying a bit."

"Please stop there, one of the commandoes said, pointing the heavy metal gun towards us. Are you any word but I was seeing many unanswered questions in her eyes but I was not in the position to answer all her questions with my heavy words.

She was about to leave and when she opened the door, a girl with the brown hairs, bright eyes, smiling lips and a small plaster on his right hand, entered the media lady paused, eyes starring at her directly.

The girl ran, jumped and hugged me tightly. My eyes were showering giving no indication to stop and she was seeing everything.

"You are really like my dad, she said cheerfully. My eyes were not astonished to see but she was the only one who survived with me. I don't know how we didn't get infected. Sometimes God plays better, even much better than our plan.

I saved everyone but didn't able to save my family, I said to the media lady, wanted to stop her. My eyes were in heavy pain and that was the day, my heart falls too, not because of the happiness but with the unbearable pain which I can't share with anyone in the world. I started my life as a stranger and ending up like a stranger but in between; I have learnt so many things and know how strangers become love when our loved ones leave us. We came alone and going alone. *We born alone with the expectation of getting new friends and then leave them with the smile on their lips and tears in their eyes. Before I say something further, my hands got down and I fell on the soft pillow reminding the moments of love and hate with the Olivia. The media lady ran towards me but it was looking like a mile for her. I left without saying anything because my heavy heart never allowed me to do so.*

I took victory over my pain and mumbled, take care of her and last breathe takes me away in the clouds. I was really embarrassed for my death but much sorry for the bad life that I gave to my family. *Sometimes we have time to understand the things around us but still, we ignore them without any further reason. Little mistakes can take us anywhere. It's our duty to correct it before it's too late. I was going with a lesson and deep pain but everything was completely over. Between the life and death, we have the opportunity to learn so many lessons and that's why we born. Maybe Olivia will meet me in new life but now I wanted to be a girl to understand the pain, tears and love inside the womb and heart of a beautiful woman.*

क्रम-सूची

भरत सा है मेरा जीवन ,
अब तो राम कृपा तुम कर दो |
मेरी सीता कुछ न कहती ,
शांत भाव से सब कुछ सेहती ,
बहुत दुखी है लव-कुश के मन ,
धन धान्य की दया तुम कर दो ,
अब तो राम कृपा तुम कर दो ।
दयानिधि है नाम तुम्हारा ,
कृपा ही करना काम तुम्हारा ,
अपनी कृपा की बारिश कर दो,
अब तो राम कृपा तुम कर दो।
मैं प्रार्थी तुम संपूरणकर्ता,
मेरी प्रार्थना पूरण कर दो ,
अब तो राम कृपा तुम दो ।

2. तुम हो

जब तेज धूप के थपेड़े चलते हो ,
तभी अचानक बादलों की छाया ,
एहसास कराती है की तूम हो |
जब मुसीबत घेर लेती है बेइंतहां ,
तब अचानक से किसी का आना ,
सहारा देना बताता है की तुम हो |
जब घिरा रहता लगातार परेशानियों में ,
तब प्यार से सहलाने का
एहसास कराता है की तुम हो |
जब भी सोता हूँ एक प्रार्थना कर के ,
कल एक नयी सुबह के इंतज़ार में ,
तब ख़्वाबों में हिम्मत बढ़ाना ,
बताता है की तुम हो।
जब भीगता हूँ अपने ही आसूओं में ,
और छलनी होता है मन ,
तब आकर मरहम का एहसास,
कराता है की तुम हो |
जब कभी समझाते थे समझता भी था ,
रोता था , नासमझ था ,
अब उस समझाइश का एहसास
कराता है की तुम हो।
अब मैं हूँ सभी आस-पास रहते है ,
लेकिन कभी प्रायः तन्हाइयों के सफर में ,

एक यात्री

ये हुनरबैज़ियाँ कब काम आएँगी |

एक यात्री

ये हुनरबैज़ियाँ कब काम आएँगी |

6. मेरी यादें

ऐ मेरी यादें मुझे याद मत आया करो !
तुम्हे जब भी याद करता हूँ,
मन कसैला हो जाता है।
ऐ मेरी यादों तुम्हारा मिजाज़
इतना कड़वा क्यों है ?
मुझे तो मेरा बचपन बड़ा
ही मीठा याद आता है !
पर तुम जब भी मेरे घर आती हो,
मेरा मिजाज़ चिड़चिड़ा कर जाती हो,
ऐ मेरी यादों मुझे याद मत आया करो।
तुम जब भी मेरे पास आती हो,
हमेशा कड़वेपन का
एहसास साथ लाती हो,
न जाने क्यों मेरा सब्र टूट जाता है ?
और मेरा सारा जीवन,
न जाने क्यों बिखर ?
ऐ मेरी यादों मुझे
याद मत आया करो।
मैं जब भी तुम्हारे साथ चलता हूँ,
मैं फिर अपने आप को खलता हूँ,
अपने एहसासों से फिसलता हूँ ,
फिर से उन्ही रास्तों पर निकलता है।
जो मुझे अपनी कमी का एहसास कराती है,

11. समय

अब तो अपने भी मुझसे कतराने लगे है,
जिन्हे मुझ तक आने में ज़माने लगे थे।
अब तो दिन में भी सपने आने लगे हैं,
इन्हे भी मुझ तक आने में ज़माने लगे हैं।
जो भी बुरा था उसे अब भुलाने लगे हैं,
दिमाग तो साफ़ था अब दिल से भी हटाने है।
रुखसत हो गए बुरे दिन अब अच्छे आने लगे हैं,
अब मेरे बच्चे भी देखकर मुझे देखकर मुस्कुराने लगे हैं।
खुशनुमा माहौल है अब कोई गम नहीं,
दिल बहुत सुकून में है अब कोई रज नहीं।
आबोहवा साफ़ है अब कोई दुश्मन नहीं,
दुःख का कोई निशान हो ऐसा कोई चमन नहीं।
कोई भी कोना नहीं है जहाँ पर अब अमन नहीं,
हर तरफ ईमान बैठा है कहीं कोई गबन नहीं।
अब उड़ान आस्मान में है कहीं बंधन नहीं,
जज़्बात अब सो गए है कहीं कोई अनबन नहीं।
बाधाएं सब दूर हो गयीं कोई भी अड़चन नहीं,
सभी से दोस्ताना है कहीं कोई दुश्मन नहीं।

12. याद रखना की मैं हूँ

जब भी थकने लगे पांव
लगने लगे सफर लम्बा,
मदद की जरुरत हो ,
याद रखना की मैं हूँ !
जब भी धुप हो कड़ी
पावों में छाले पड़ने लगे,
सीना धधक उठे चीत्कार से,
याद रखना की मैं हूँ !
संघर्ष बढ़ रहे हों
जीवन का रास्ता कठिन हो,
एक पग भी बढ़ाना कठिन हो,
याद रखना की मैं हूँ।
सभी ने छोड़ा हो साथ
कोई न पकड़ रहा हो हाथ,
सहारे की हो तलाश,
याद रखना की मैं हूँ !
सब चले जाएँ छोड़ कर
बैठ जाए तुम से मुँह मोड़कर,
यदि हो किसी का इंतज़ार,
तो याद रखना की मैं हूँ !
सुख में मिल ही जाते है सब
दुःख में काम आते हैं रब,
जब आये यादों की बारात,

16. एतबार

हद से ज़्यादा
किसी का एतबार मत करना !
कोई मन से मिल जाये तो ठीक
नहीं तो इंतज़ार मत करना।
ये जो चीज़ है
जिसे मोहब्बत कहते है,
इसमें कोई राज़दार मत रखना
मिल जाये तो ठीक
नहीं तो अपने दिल को वज़नदार मत करना।
राह में कोई जो मिल जाये,
तो मिलने से पहले
थोड़ी दरार रखना !
ये ही डुबाएगी बीच मझदारों में,
हाथों में अपने पतवार रखना।
ये है न जो चाहने वाले,
बीच में छोड़ना शोक है इनका !
अपने दिल को इनके लिए
खबरदार रखना !
ये जो छोड़ भी जाये तो,
जो काम यही इनका
अपनी दुआओं से अपना दिल वफादार रखना।
ये जो मिलते हैं
जुबानी खंजर चलाने वाले,

इनके लिए अपनी जुबान को धारदार रखना !
ये लोग है जो बुरा ही कहते हैं,
इनका भी तमाशा बना सको
ऐसा एक वफादार रखना।

20. ये किसी का न हुआ

ये है मेरा ,वह तुम्हारा
हम सभी का न हुआ
इसको ढूंढा,उसको ढूंढा
मन कभी भी न छुआ
साथ में इसके भी बैठा
साथ में उसके भी बैठा
अपना नहीं कोई हुआ।
मैं गया इस रास्ते पर,
मैं गया उस रास्ते पर,
सभी रास्ते तंग मिले,
दोस्त न अपना मिला।
मैंने देखा हर तरफ
बस खुदी को नहीं देखा !
खुद के भीतर मैंने झाँका,
मैं ही खुद को न मिला।
चल रहा था मैं जिस पथ पर
वह पथ भी मेरा न हुआ !
फूल भी सब शूल हो गए
कंटक भरा ये मन हुआ।
अब न जाने कब रिक्त होगा,
मन भरा जो सालों से,
ब्रंह की आवाज़ ने मेरे मन को छुआ !
कुछ गया है बहुत कुछ शेष है,

कुछ नया अब होने वाला,
ब्रम्हांड में कुछ तो हुआ है।

कुछ नया अब होने वाला,
ब्रम्हांड में कुछ तो हुआ है।

मनोरथ पूर्ण होते हम सभी के
वर सभी हो जाते हैं अविनाश
जब कहती हो तुम
कर सकता हूँ मैं ! कर सकता हूँ मैं !
हम सभी ऋणी है तुम्हारे
धन्य हूँ पाया तुम्ही को
तुम सुरक्षित देविय कृपा से
हो गए सब सौभाग्य वासी
जब कहती हो तुम
कर सशक्त हूँ मैं ! कर सकता हूँ मैं !

25. अधिकार

न झुका हूँ ,न झुकूंगा
न रुका हूँ ,न रूकूंगा
न कभी नतमस्त था मैं,
न ही याचना मैं करूंगा।
जो मिला है अधिकार मेरा,
जो मिलेगा आभार होगा,
अब ना होगी याचना कोई,
अब न होगी प्रार्थना कोई,
अधिकार मेरा मुझको मिलेगा।
भूत से वर्तमान तक,
यह विरासत सम्पूर्ण मेरी,
अधिकार मुझको न मिला तो,
रणक्षेत्र का संधान होगा।
भीष्म बनकर तप कर चूका हूँ,
द्रोपदी सम चीर का बलिदान देकर,
कृष्ण है अब साथ मेरे,
पार्थ का गांडीव बनकर,
इस धरा पर मैं गिरूंगा,
अधिकार अपना मैं वरूँगा,
सम्मान अपना मैं धरूंगा।।

29. माँ हो तुम

मुझे परेशान देखकर , मेरे मन को टटोलना,
यह हुनर सिर्फ तुझमे है क्योंकि माँ हो तुम।
आज भी मेरे बचपने पर खिलखिलाती हो,
और साहिल हो जाती हो क्योंकि माँ हो तुम।
अपनी परेशानियों को हमेशा भूल जाती हो,
मैं जब परेशान होता हूँ क्योंकि माँ हो तुम।
मुसीबतों और परेशानियों में शांत रहकर,
औरों से छिपकर सहारा बनती हो क्योंकि माँ हो तुम।
सभी के बीच रहती हो पक्षपात भी करती हो,
डांटती हो , प्यार भी करती हो क्योंकि माँ हो तुम।
ये अवस्था और शरीर भी कमज़ोर है,
पर पूरे ज़ोर से हिम्मत बढाती हो क्योंकि माँ हो तुम।
तुम्हारा आँचल एक छत का एहसास कराता है,
सभी आँधियों से बचती हो क्योंकि माँ हो तुम।।

30. रमता रमन

मैं रहा रमता रमन,
साफ़ थे मेरे आचरण,
फिर भी साद मैं छला ही गया।
मैं सदा वैट वृक्ष सा था,
वे सभी अमर बेल बक बन गए,
फिर भी मैं सदा छांव देता,
प्रत्येक क्षण मरता गया।
मैं सदा ही नीव पत्थर,
मैं कभी छत सा सहारा,
फिर कभी दीवार भी था,
और वे उसमे रहने वाले,
प्रति पल मुझे खोले रहे।
मैं चला सब साथ लेकर,
मैं चला जग साथ लेकर,
फिर भी सफर में अकेला,
हाथ खली साथ खली,
मैं जाग्रत ता उम्र था,
वे सदा सुख सुख सोते रहे।
अब नव लक्ष्य मेरे,
अब नए शस्त्र धारण किये हैं,
अब नया संधान होगा,
अब नहीं स्व सहानुभूति,
नकारात्मक अब त्यागना है,

34. परिंदे

सुहाने स्वप्न अब आने लगे हैं,
कुस्वप्न अब सारे जाने लगे हैं,
शुभ शगुन का हो रहा आगाज़ अब तो
मेरे घर के परिंदे अब परवाज़ पर जाने लगे हैं।
रूठे हुए जो थे वो अब मिलने आने लगे हैं,
कतरा कर जाने वाले हाथों को अब मिलाने लगे हैं,
भरा रहता है आजकल आँगन मेरा
जब से बादल खुशियों के मेरे घर पर मंडराने लगे हैं।
पीर और दरवेश मेरे दर पर आने लगे हैं,
बधाईयां देने वाले आँगन खटखटाने लगे हैं,
भर गया है रोशनाईयों से अब मेरा घर
सोने चांदी के तकिये सर के सिरहाने लगे है।
कदम खुद व खुद मंदिर को जाने लगे हैं,
ताल बजने लगे हैं घंटे भी बजाने लगे है,
सौभाग्य पर इतराने लगा हूँ मैं
मनुज की बात क्या अब देव भी अपनाने लगे हैं।
बुरी यादों से अब बाहर आने लगे हैं,
रकीबों को भी अब नश्वर चुभने लगे हैं,
अब तो सभी फासले से मिलते हैं
जिन्हे आने में ज़माने लगे हैं।
में जिन्हे सारी उम्र पालता रहा,
वो सपने अब पूरे होने लगे हैं,
में उन्हें रोज़ देखता हूँ

मेरे बच्चे अब बड़े होने लगे हैं।

जो मिले आभार होगा।
आइये स्वागत तो कर लें,
जो आ रहा बाँहों में भर लें।
मन के आँगन आनंद घर लें,
अब न कोई ताप होगा
हर तरफ उल्लास होगा।

39. कृष्णा-याचना

क्या क्या दे पाओगे,
जो माँगा वो मिला नहीं,
तुमसे जब भी लेने आया,
तुमको सदा निसहाय पाया।
ये सुना था तुम सहाय सबके,
तुम्ही सभी का पालन करते।
जो भी सद्भाव से आता,
हर विचार उसका सच हो जाता,
मेरी बारी तुम्हे क्या हो जाता,
तुम्हे सदा निसहाय पता।
ये सुना तुम पूर्ण करता
मनकामना के सम्पूर्ण करता
हर कार्य के करता धरता
विघ्न विनाशक विघ्नो के हर्ता
मेरी समझ में कुछ नहीं आता
तुम्हे सदा निसहाय पता
मैं तुम्हे किस तरह ध्याऊँ
मैं तुम्हे किस तरह मनाऊं
अपना वर यथार्थ में पाऊं
कोनसा पथ मैं अपनाऊं
मैं भी उच्च सफल हो जाऊं
तुम्हे सदा सहाय पाऊं
तुम्हारा निज सेवक बन जाऊं

तेरे बिन नहीं रहा जाता।
अब तो कृष्णा मेरे पास आयो,
दिव्य दर्शन तुम कराओ,
ऐसा सम्भन्ध तुम से बनाऊं,
जब भी बुलाऊँ पास पाऊं।
अब तो कृष्णा तुम ऐसा कर दो,
उदास मन को खुशियों से भर दो।
मैं भी आला गीत गाऊं,
कृष्णा-कृष्णा की रट लगाऊं।।

43. कृष्णा-जीवन

तुम सदा परदे में रहते,
मुस्कान को अधरों पे धरते,
बंसी की तुम तान करते,
गुंजायमान आकाश करते,
हे कृष्णा! तुम हो हमारे।
घंटों का है नाद होता,
भक्तों से संवाद होता,
पंडों का भी साथ होता,
आनंद से अट्टहास होता,
हे कृष्णा ! तुम हो हमारे।
आलय है सबसे निराला,
राधा का है साथ आला,
यषोदा और नंद लाला,
चाहने पर सब मिलने वाला,
तुम सभी का ध्यान धरते,
हे कृष्णा ! तुम हो हमारे।
गोकुल का तू रहने वाला,
मथुरा में आकर डेरा डाला,
कंस को नष्ट कर डाला,
संसार को तुमने सम्भाला,
तुम सभी विघ्नों को हरते,
हे कृष्णा ! तुम हो हमारे।
हम सभी तुम्हारे पास आते,

47. खुद से ही करना होता है

जो करना हो वो होता है,
खुद करना हो तब होता है,
जब करना हो तब करना है.
लेकिन तुमको खुद करना है।
खुद के मरे ही स्वर्ग दिखता है,
जब तू करता है तब मिलता,
जब मैदान में तू निकलता है,
जो भी करना वो होता है,
खुद करना हो तब होता है,
सबसे रिश्ता तब चलता है,
खुद अपने ज़ख्मों को तू सिलता है,
सबसे मन तब मिलता है,
जब अपने मन से तू मिलता है,
सारा गुलशन तब खिलता है,
हर आँगन मानव मिलता है,
जो करना हो वो होता है,
खुद करना हो तब होता है।
वो भी तुझसे तब मिलता है,
जब अपने घर में तू मिलता है,
तेरा तुझको तब मिलता है,
सबका सबको सब मिलता है,
जो भी करना हो तब होता है,

खुद करना हो तब होता है,
तेरे मन का तब होता है।
जो पाना हो मन बोता है,
पौधा बढ़ता फल मिलता हैं,
आज नहीं तो कल मिलता है,
जो भी करना हो तब होता है,
खुद करना हो तब होता है।
अपने आप को क्यों खोता है,
क्यों खोने पर तू खोता है,
फसल का मालिक वो होता है,
जो उसको खुद बोता है।
मिट्टी होने पर रोता है,
जो भी करना वो होता है,
खुद करना हो तो होता है।

फैसला मिट चूका कभी का,
ये ज़मीन , वो आस्मां तक
जहाँ भी देखूं मैं वहां तक,
तय शिखर को छु चूका हूँ।
ये ज़मीन वो चाँद तारे,
सारे हो गए हैं हमारे,
मेरे साथ ही हैं सारे,
बाँहों को अपनी पसारे,
दिल तक सभी के जा चूका हूँ,
तय शिखर को छु चूका हूँ।

WHAT WOULD SHE LOOK LIKE?

LONGDISTANCE LOVE REQUIRES US TO HAVE A DIFFERENT IMAGE OF THE PERSON WE LOVE. WE HAVE NO IDEA HOW THE PERSON WILL SPEAK. BECAUSE THE ONLY THING THAT BRINGS PEOPLE TOGETHER IS THE EXCHANGE OF WORDS. THERE ARE MANY QUESTIONS RUNNING THROUGH A PERSON HEAD THAT COULD ONLY BE ANSWERED IF THE PERSON MET HIS/HER LOVE.

Aakhen talash rhi thi kuch palo ko

Aaj wo mere darwaje pe dastak dene lage hai

Zindgi mai saki ke alava bhi apna mann hum kisi se lagane chale hai

Tasveer se lekar ro ba ro hone ka safar jaam leke humne kaat lia

Or log sochte hai ke saharab sirf mekhane mai milti hai

Aashiqo se puchoo kitnaa sabar or ishq milane ke baad ek katra sharab banti hai

Or aaj Apni zindagi ko uski aakhon se nasha karane ja rha hu mai

YOU ARE AN ANGEL

Tu kisi pari se kam nhi hai

Tere husan ka jadu mujhpe har roz hota hai

Jab tu na nikle ghr se toh pure sheher mai andhera hota hai

Or wo aakhon se jo tu roz nasha karati hai na mujhe

Us surror ka pta sirf mere dil ko hota hai

Or jab sharab ko chhuta tha toh kha makha badnam tha

Zamana kya jane asli nasha bin chuyee teri aadaon se hota hai

Or jab tu chattt par paas bulkar ,zara sa muskurakar ,nazre milakar ,palke jhuka kar ,mujhme samaya karti hai na

Uska ehesas mujhe nhi pure aaasman ko hota hai

Or sachai sun paas baith muskura

Tere husn ka jadu mujhpe nhi pure sheher par hota hai

Nikalti ghr se tu nhi hai or andhera pure sheher mai hota hai....

BETRAYAL

WHEN PERSON CAME ACROSS THE BETRAYAL FROM HER OR HIS LOVE. THAT TIME A PERSON SPENDS ALONE IN HIS ROOM AND MAKES HIMSELF ISOLATED FROM THE WORLD. THE ROOM OR WALL HAD THOSE FEELING AS HUMAN HAS, THEY COULD TELL HER/ HIM THE PAIN AND HOW DARKEST DREAM HAD FORGED HIM/ HER IN THE LOOP OF HAPPINESS AND SADNESS.

Humko dur bhejnaa bhale khwaab hoga tera

Magar humara dur janaa lagbhag shraap hoga tera

Chalee jayegee yuhi khii durr , mera kamraa hi hai itna mashurr, sirhane m sir rkh usne har drd dekhe h mere, tu itna kreeb hoke bhi na jaan payi or mere takhiye ne har ek aasu sokhe hai mere

Shayad Kisi or rishtedaar se rishte nibhane lgi ho

Yaa pano pe se humari shyahi mitane lagi ho

Bhale Mai musafir hu , nashe ka aadi hu sahiba

Kabhi durr saalo m milunga toh tujhse puchnga zaroor

Ke wo gardan pe tha kiska nishan sahiba

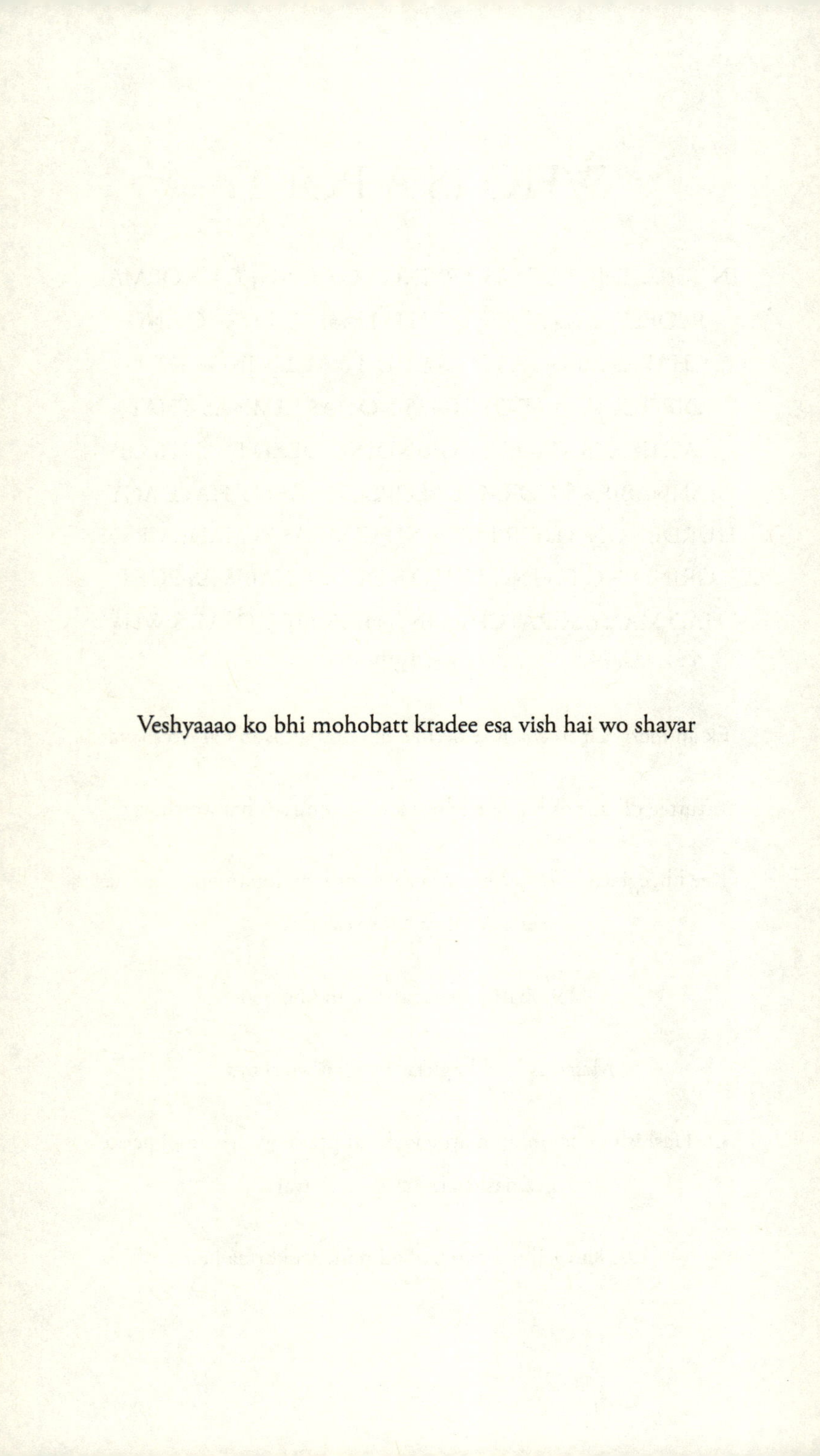

Veshyaaao ko bhi mohobatt kradee esa vish hai wo shayar

LONG TIME TALK

AFTER FALLING APART. THE DIVERGE RIVER HAS ONCE AGAIN CONJOINT. PATH THAT HAD CHANGED THAT PATH HAD ONCE AGAIN CROSSED EACH OTHER. THOUGHTS HAVE LITTLE CHANGED IN IT BECAUSE THEY HAD TRAVELLED DIFFERENT CURVES AND PATH.

She:- Ye aakhon ke neeche kesa ghera hai

Me:- Tu jo kajal lagati thi usi ka phera hai

She :- ye aakhen lal or is nami ka ilaaj kya hai

Me:- Lal toh ishq hai or nami ka ilaj toh saki ka chera hai

She :- mekhane mai waqt kuch jyada zaya nhi krte ho?

ME:- Bewafa ho tum meetha bolke zeher pilate ho ,or wo kadva hi pilati h lekin ishq pilati hai

Dard walo ke sare assu peejati hai , uski aakhon mai har dard wale ka chera hai

Ab btao kese na kahe ke is drd ka ilaj saki ka chera h

Pass rhekar izhaar karwana hai toh bhi thk hai

Lori sunatee toh zyada acha rheta

Humari gazale hi gungunani hai toh bhi thk hai

Talab ke paas milne aate toh aacha rheta

Rulake agar samandar hi banwana hai toh bhi thik hai ..

SHE DOESNT CARE

WHEN SOMEONE DOESN'T CARE OR ACCEPT THE
FEELING OF OTHER PERSON. PERSON CAME AT THE
POINT TOLERANCE AND SHOW SOMEONE THAT HE/
SHE HAS SOLVENCY OF WORD FOR OTHER.

Tu itnaaa kaam kr , thodi si jaan le magar jaan toh leee

Dard kya h dil kaa teri bewafai hi toh h , ab nhi krenge mohobat

kaam ka h dil ise kaam toh lee

Or har sham sharab se zakhmon ki baat karata hu

Tere diye zakhmon jiti sharab nhi mere ps thodee zakham apne

pass toh lee

Or Bhe gyaa lahuu kya kre manjha hi kanch ka tha

Beshakkk mai ashique tha magar banda mai kaam ka thaa

Ek khanjar saa seene mai utar dee

dekhh nikl rhi jaan , meri jaan thodii aah toh lee..

DU MÊME AUTEUR

Le Frein et l'Aiguillon. Éloquence musicale et nombre oratoire (XVIe-XVIIIe siècle), Paris, Classiques Garnier, coll. « Renaissance latine », n° 2, 2013.

Érasme, *Les Adages*, édition bilingue français-latin, Paris, Les Belles Lettres, 2011 (traduction des adages 3601 à 3700).

En collaboration

Joachim Burmeister, *Poétique musicale suivi de David Chytraeus – De la Musique*, traduction, introduction, notes et lexique par Agathe Sueur et Pascal Dubreuil, Paris, Rhuthmos, 2017.

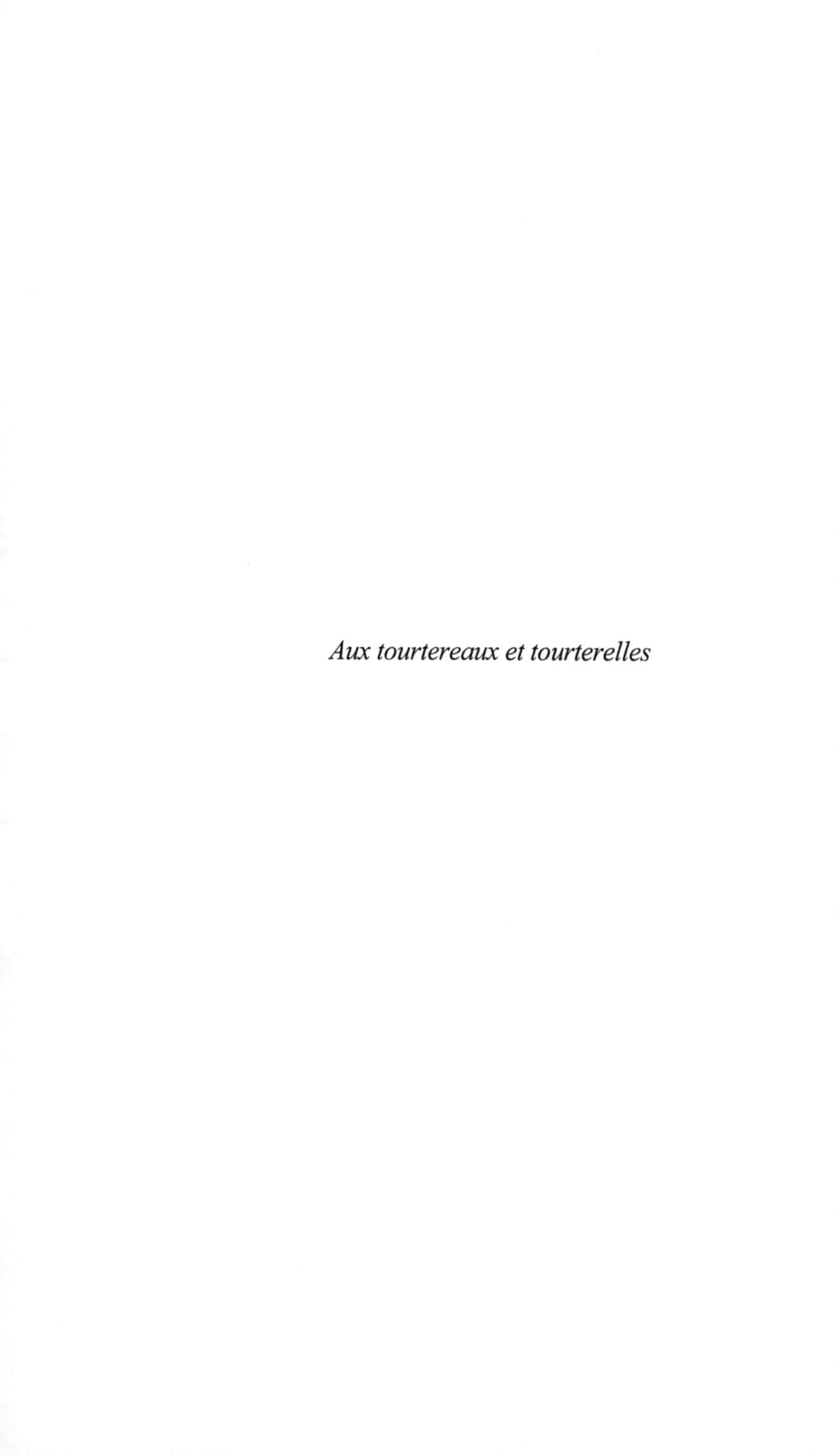

Aux tourtereaux et tourterelles

l'aiguille que quelques miettes des festivités d'un grand mariage, célébré avec tambours et ronflantes traversées de la ville : *Dorothea von Dänemark* épousant en 1561 *Wilhelm der Jüngere*, duc et futur prince de Brunswick-Lunebourg. Loin des ors sonnants et trompettants, Joachim vivotait dans son obscure demeure, s'usait les yeux sur de rares tissus, et quand il prit femme en la personne de Margarete Soltau, fille de marchand (toujours de ces maudits marchands), il dut se demander à quoi servirait d'égrener année après année des rejetons, fruit de leur pieux mariage, à qui ni les harengs ni les princes ne voudraient apporter de l'or.

Mais en frais réformé spirituellement nourri des leçons de D. M. L., Docteur Martin Luther, dont il avait vu passer un jour l'effigie, fort peu perlée, sur une gravure tachée de graisse, en jeune réformé qui se gardait respectueusement des sirènes de la bière rousse, en réformé pointilleux qui ne souffrait pas outre mesure de rouler son rocher de Sisyphe, puisqu'il ignorait jusqu'au nom de Sisyphe, il fit ce que lui-même pouvait faire, c'est-à-dire ce que la Bible commandait, désormais en allemand, bien qu'on l'eût déjà entendue du temps où elle parlait latin ; et à défaut de réussir à faire croître et multiplier l'or, il fit croître et multiplier une famille : le premier-né fut un garçon qu'il appela, fier et résolu, Joachim.

Je ne parlerai pas des autres enfants qui suivirent Joachim fils, on a assez glosé sur eux, vous les avez vus en rang d'oignons, défilant poliment dans les notices biographiques : Anton, qui fut cantor à l'église Saint-Michel de Lunebourg ; Frantz, qui fut organiste à l'église St-Lambert à Lunebourg ; Georg, qui fut recteur de l'école Saint-Michel à Lunebourg ; Joannes, qui fut couronné poète lauréat du Saint Empire, qui publia, excusez du peu, des parodies sacrées et christianisées des pourtant vertes et truculentes épigrammes de Martial, et qui fut un frère d'autant plus fidèle, qu'il était un cousin de Joachim, comme le révèlent les plus récentes et scrupuleuses notules de telle société de philologie néolatine. Passons aussi sur les noms avortés et autres filles absentes, mort-nées ou tristes fruits de fausses couches.

Ce que l'on sait de son enfance, c'est-à-dire pas grand-chose, le voici : il fut un enfant doux, à la parole rare, qui dans les premiers temps n'eut de plus grand plaisir que celui d'observer, tapi dans un recoin, son père inlassablement occupé à trier perles, fils, soie, or, satin, dans le modeste homéotéleutes, allitérations et autres assonances, accumulations, le tout bardé, comme un rôti de Pentecôte, de ces noms de métiers qui, sans doute possible, raviraient un public conquis sans avoir à combattre. *Stat fullo, phrygio, aurifex, lanarius…* et la pittoresque procession bas-latine des marchands se pressa en son théâtre intérieur comme à la porte de Mégadore, où *d'abord se tient le foulon, le brodeur, l'orfèvre, le marchand de laine…* et le maître sut qu'il triompherait.

Mais n'étant point de ces inventeurs qui arborent sourire satisfait et vulgaire à la première idée venue, il affina et raffina son petit piège à garnements, si bien que le jour dit, les lutins bas-saxons virent l'œil du maître pétiller plus que de coutume au moment de commencer la leçon de grammaire quotidienne, avec au menu pour ce jour, déclinaisons, déclinaisons, déclinaisons. *Ex abrupto* on déclina *fullo* : *fullo, fullo, fullonem, fullonis, fulloni, fullone.* On déclina *phrygio* : *phrygio, phrygio, phrygionem, phrygionis, phry-gioni, phrygione.* On déclina, *etcetera.* Et lorsqu'il sentit l'attention de son auditoire vacillante, sur le point de s'abîmer dans un chahut diabolique digne des ténèbres papistes, le *magister ludi* se tut et d'un air mystérieux disposa en silence sur sa grande table de curieuses petites boîtes. Et le jeu commença : les fringants humanisticules eurent à choisir, rangées en chacune d'elles, de petites perles de verre colorées qu'ils devaient associer dûment, une à une, à chacune des figures dont le nom (à défaut de l'identité) venait d'être décliné. Au *fullo*, le foulon, revint la petite perle rouge sombre, parce qu'il foule le raisin gorgé de soleil (et certes celui-là ne se trouve point en Basse-Saxe). Au *phrygio*, le brodeur de perles, revint la petite perle irisée, et lors les lutins se tournèrent vers le lutin Joachim : *Phrygio est pater Joachimi !* Ainsi, avec patience et passion, ils égrenèrent et reconnurent déclinaisons, couleurs, métiers, et leurs pères, et leurs oncles, voisins, cousins, auréolés des généreuses sonorités latines. Et ce faisant, pour la plus discrète satisfaction du maître, ils apprirent leurs premiers vers de Plaute – huit vers, Monsieur. *Stat fullo, phrygio, aurifex, lanarius*, rouge sombre, nacre, or brillant, beige ; *Caupones, patagiarii, indusiarii,* les cabaretiers, faiseurs de franges, fabricants de chemise, marron, blanc brillant, blanc mat ; *Flammearii, violarii, carinarii,* les teinturiers en couleur de flammes, en violet, en brou de noix ; je m'arrête là, Monsieur, et vous épargne volontiers le détail des cordonniers, savetiers, teinturiers spécialisés dans la pourpre ou le mauve, marchands de lacets ou de ceintures, qui vous

Vérité d'amour à n'en pas douter. Là est le paradis des roses, là s'emparent de vous les fragrances enchanteresses de milliers de roses, rouges, orangées, blanches, incarnates, noires, jaunes, violacées, pourpres, *etcetera, etcetera*. Ah Monsieur, quelle heureuse surprise pour Joachim, et aussi bien pour tout voyageur qui découvre en ces lieux que pays des Vandales peut rimer avec pastorale.

Vous revoilà donc à la porte de Kröpelin et ses promesses de roses, mais – ne vous agacez point, je vous prie – il vous faut gagner à nouveau, en toute hâte, la porte Saint-Pierre, car c'est de là que vous déambulerez dans les ruelles, passages, rues et venelles de Rostock pour connaître en son tréfonds la cité ; cité qui, sachez-le, se compose de trois parties, la première, la deuxième et la troisième. Et pour commencer, l'ancienne, à l'est, au pied de Saint-Pierre donc, arborant sa vieille place, *forum vetus*, et son vieux marché où les paysans se pressent pour faire leur commerce de bois, de charbon, d'orge, après quoi, plutôt que de regagner *illico* leurs rustiques pénates, ils font la sieste en cette place même, Monsieur ; et après la partie ancienne vient, plus à l'ouest, la médiane où loge la fleur de la bourgeoisie dans d'élégantes maisons ornées de leurs petits pans de brique rouge et pignons lorgnant vers la place centrale, *forum medium*. Et c'est en cette place qu'est sise la mairie coiffée de ses sept tourelles, du haut desquelles une troupe d'oiseaux de mer plutôt gloutons que réformés attend chaque jour la fin du marché pour piller plutôt que glaner une roborative subsistance : c'est là que vous ferez journellement vos emplettes, Monsieur, si vous voulez vivre à Rostock. Enfin, plus à l'ouest encore, vous vous hâterez vers la partie nouvelle de la ville, le *forum Lupuli*, la place au houblon, *lupulus*, aussi appelée la place aux chevaux, parce que les maquignons y font commerce en de certains jours ; et encore appelée, Monsieur, le *forum Latinum*, parce que se dressent alentour, sobres et doctes, les collèges où s'enseignent les humanités, en langues grecque et latine.

Et Monsieur l'érudit de Rostock, intarissable, poursuit ses comptes en ses tablettes, égrenant inlassablement ses chiffres et ses mots : c'est que, figurez-vous bien cela, Monsieur, Rostock compte plus de mille constructions, maisons et édifices, environ cent quarante rues, dont vous aurez plaisir à savoir que certaines tirent leurs noms des portes de la ville vers lesquelles elles dardent leurs pavés, la rue de pierre, la rue *qu'il n'est point de rythme dans la pure continuité uniforme : mais qu'au contraire, le rythme naît d'une distinction et percussion à intervalles égaux et parfois variés ; qu'on peut l'observer dans les gouttes de pluie qui tombent* (et Dieu sait s'il pleut à Rostock), *parce que celles-ci sont distinguées par des intervalles, tandis qu'on ne le peut dans un fleuve qui se précipite d'un flot uni* (et Dieu sait que la Warnow est un fort menu Danube). On sait cela, Monsieur, parce que l'étudiant Joachim Burmeister obtint un prix *maxima cum laude* pour le commentaire qu'il fit de ce texte : commentaire aujourd'hui perdu, modeste trace effacée par le temps. Commentaire brillant, à en croire les autorités des Roses, et rien d'étonnant à cela, Monsieur. C'est que du rythme, depuis sa prime enfance, Joachim avait bien plus que des rudiments, ayant si souvent écouté les discours de l'orgue, la conversation familière des moulins à vent ou à eau ; ayant si souvent, aussi, observé les doigts de son père virevoltant sur les étoffes : car en ce temps il n'est point de motif brodé qui ne cache un rythme pour l'œil, Monsieur.

1593 fut une année intense – je dis 1593, Monsieur, parce que vous êtes lettré, parce que vous avez lu et qu'il me prend envie de singer pour quelques instants les grands mages du récit d'histoire, les magiciens apothicaires et maîtres brasseurs de la liqueur historique, passionnés de millésimes. Voyez-les qui, savants en l'art de pilloter çà et là, abeilles voraces autant qu'industrieuses, collectent, récoltent sans répit faits et dates, modestes nectars, pour en faire aussitôt un miel bâtard autant que bigarré – *toutes fleurs* –, qu'ils rehaussent en secret de quelques épices caléfactives ou dormitives ; voyez-les qui, savants en l'art de concasser, moudre, broyer, piler, distiller, jettent leur dévolu sur les grands ou menus événements égrenés par la petite chronique, les candides annales, les braves et dociles registres, pour bientôt les laisser infuser, filtrer et fermenter. Ah, Monsieur, admirez-les, nos fiers abstracteurs de quintessence, qui maintenant plastronnent et se font forts de vous vendre au meilleur prix l'esprit-de-telle-année – 476, 800, 1453, 1515, 1648, 1789, 1793, laquelle souhaitez-vous ? en poudre bienfaisante, qu'on recommande à la mémoire ? ou en liqueur, dans sa petite fiole, bienheureux viatique pour les esprits qui, voyageant loin et battant la campagne, veulent ménager leur monture ? Ah, qu'on se le dise, et qu'on s'en gargarise à gorge déployée, de ces dates symboliques, de ces dates emblématiques, de ces dates substantifiques. Ma foi, tous ces

non un monstre, cet homme, entouré de trois
compagnons aux mines indécises à force de
humer l'air épais, poisseux et putride, est un
alchimiste d'un tout autre genre que celui auquel
vous a habitué la bonne petite imagerie dans le
goût flamand, qui brode à plaisir sur son ermite
grisonnant, solitaire comme Jérôme en sa grotte,
encombré de cornues, alambics, creusets et livres
de cabale ; l'alchimiste dont je parle, Monsieur,
transforme quant à lui, non pas le plomb en or,
mais le poisson en colle, l'os de bœuf en lamelle,
et le plomb en tuyau. Et Burmeister, samedi après
samedi, l'œil pailleté de joie à mesure que son
nez suffoque, jamais ne se lasse d'observer les
curieux échafauds, tréteaux, sommiers, panneaux
de toutes tailles qui inlassablement s'entassent là,
puis peu à peu s'ordonnent comme en procession, en vue de quelque mystérieux rituel ; et
scintillant, fredonnant, vibrionnant parmi vilebre-
quins, équerres, compas, scies et rabots, le regard
du sémillant visiteur parfois se perd, se fixe puis
s'absorbe dans la contemplation de certaines
petites boîtes, menus tiroirs et simples tirettes
moulurées qui bientôt, il le sait, seront parés de
ces noms précieux et ambrés, à eux donnés par
l'obscur artisan, dans le secret de l'atelier. Et
déjà, comme évoqués par quelque philtre d'outre-
monde, ces noms s'égrènent et sonnent en silence,

de leur son d'airain épuré, pour le plaisir de l'initié : mixture, bourdon, régale, cromorne s'invitent en son esprit, et plus d'un soir y dansent une ineffable sarabande nocturne.

J'y viens, Monsieur, j'y viens : notre alchimiste vexe-narines a nom Heinrich Glowatz, bon bourgeois de Rostock, qui aux harengs, aux perles, aux onguents, a préféré les orgues, oui, les orgues. Je dis les orgues par manière d'honorer le féminin pluriel, car en fait d'orgue on ne lui connaît que celui-ci, livré en 1593 à l'église Sainte-Marie de Rostock. Un facteur d'orgue, ce Glowatz, artisan, maître ès métaux et bois – louez-le à bon compte autant que vous voudrez –, mais avant tout marchand, Monsieur, comme tout bon bourgeois de Rostock, et à ce titre aussi bien expert en chiffres, comptes et tablettes : pensez un peu, quel orgue que celui-ci, pavané de ses chiffres, cinq mille florins de coût pour trente-neuf jeux, quatorze soufflets, trois claviers ; quel orgue, égrenant la lente suite et procession de ses jeux, c'est à savoir le grand orgue, avec six jeux, Monsieur, principal large, mixture, cymbale, bourdon 16 pieds, octave 8 pieds, superoctave 4 pieds ; un positif pectoral de douze jeux, régale-violon, cromorne 8 pieds, sedetz 1 pied, sifflet, superoctave 2 pieds, flûte à bec, régale 8 pieds, rien, sinon le mot *phrygio*, d'auguste renommée. Elle assista de loin, pensive et fière, à la cérémonie, suivit la procession des lauréats à pas menus, comme une petite souris dont le froid rosit le museau, toujours bien accompagnée par les deux fringants et délicieux larrons. Point de fête, en ce cas, Monsieur, qui ne finisse à la taverne, dans le joyeux concert boisé des chopines. L'on but, l'on rit ; et soudain la mère semble fatiguée, séchée, recroquevillée ; elle demande à Joannes de la raccompagner à leur logis, prie Joachim de ne point s'inquiéter. Elle sort, pareille à une feuille de tremble à sa dernière heure, par une nuit de novembre. Le silence se fait, chacun, à la table contrariée, entend en soi la pluie, glaciale, qui tombe drue sur la cité des Roses. Mais soudain, ô surprise, la mère est là, bien là, de nouveau là, et cette fois elle est immense, touche presque au plafond, drapée dans un magnifique drap brodé, toge improvisée, elle est là, un bonnet carré sur le chef, elle jubile, telle une papesse des fous, et dit d'une voix nimbée d'or, bien qu'un brin hésitante : *Magister est filius meus !* Puis elle se tourne vers Anton, son autre fils ici présent, et claironne : *Tu quoque, mi fili ! Volo te in Academiâ Rosarum studere !* Alors les deux petits yeux de la mère, clairs comme la Baltique en hiver sous le ciel délavé, brillent comme jamais, et les larmes perlent aux yeux de Joachim. Pensez un peu, Monsieur, quelle fierté pour une mère. Et bientôt, la douce Margarete à la voix rauque, l'humble Marguerite à la voix douce, s'incline, sa toge se fend, et Joannes apparaît, portant sa très chère tante juchée sur ses épaules, sa tante dont il fut le professeur en langue étrange pour un soir. Le cousin lui aussi a gagné sa place à Rostock, et il ne reste à l'aîné qu'à veiller sur ses chers Dioscures de cadets, par son autorité de professeur.

Mais laissons là les Burmeister et leur petite légende, leur petit rêve familier, et parlons un peu, Monsieur. Que savez-vous au juste de ce métier de professeur, auquel Burmeister s'est vu condamné à perpétuité par les édiles enfarinés ? – Hier ou aujourd'hui, peu importe, c'est égal, rien n'a changé, je vous rassure. Savez-vous ce que c'est que d'être précepteur classique en classe seconde à l'école sénatoriale de Rostock, dite aussi école inférieure ou triviale ? Savez-vous, enfin – venons-en au point, Monsieur – ce que c'est que Sisyphe ? À Rostock, à Lunebourg, à Vierzon, peu importe, vous dis-je. *La poussière de l'école. In pulvere scholastico*, comme le dit le très cher, le très docte docteur Joannes Bacmeister dans sa petite complainte funèbre, comme l'ont dit, répété, ressassé les Allemands pendant deux siècles, deux l'ancienne Rome. Il songe, aussi. Il songe, plus d'une fois, le regard absorbé au loin, contemplant de certaines petites fleurs blanches sur le perron de Sainte-Marie. Car il est en son cœur une corde secrète cassée, que ni luth, ni clavicorde, ni tourterelle ne sauraient lui faire oublier, et qui se nomme rameau d'or. Eh oui, Monsieur, vous le savez, je vous l'ai dit, le beau rameau d'or – entendez, les secrets de la théorie musicale, le grimoire du seigneur Henricus Brucaeus, docteur et pythie de son état – est enfui. Mais voici qu'un matin, sur ce même parvis de Sainte-Marie, deux colombes se posent devant Joachim et l'observent de leurs petits yeux tendres. Il lève la tête, son regard se fixe : en cet instant précis, Burmeister a compris.

Burmeister a compris, mais pas vous, Monsieur, je le crains, égaré que vous êtes dans cet obscur cabinet de curiosités où frayent colombes, petites fleurs blanches et rameau d'or. Et vous vous dites, peut-être, que me voilà à mon tour égaré dans le dédale de mon petit bavardage, que la fée Mythologie m'ensorcelle et me fait désirer, ô désastre, d'être sphinge, débitant paroles énigmatiques aussi bien que cryptiques. Rassurez-vous, il n'en est rien, je n'ai point ce désir. Et pour preuve, souffrez que je vous explique par quelles subtilités de la grâce divine un manuscrit pétri de chiffres et mathématique peut se métamorphoser en petite branche aux feuilles brillantes, en rameau d'or. Vous saurez donc, Monsieur, qu'au siècle seizième en l'ère de notre Seigneur la musique se pensait et se divisait en deux parties, la pratique et la théorique ; qu'en la pratique se rangeaient toutes choses de chair et de son à l'usage des musiciens, chanteurs, cantors, tous artisans soufflant, tâtant, palpant, touchant cordes, claviers, fabriquant de ces vibrations aériennes qui poignent et émeuvent les corps et les cœurs, avant que d'atteindre les âmes. Vous saurez, ensuite, qu'en la théorique se pressaient toutes choses d'esprit et d'abstraction, à savoir processions de chiffres, tables et théorèmes accompagnés de leurs démonstrations, scolies et corollaires, s'avançant tous, comme le veut la coutume, à *la manière géométrique, more geometrico*, et tous adoubés par les anciens maîtres, Pythagore, Euclide, Boèce et leurs émules. Ah, Monsieur, que de splendeurs, que de beautés d'esprit en la musique appelée théorique, par la grâce de laquelle vous saurez par exemple – pour cette fois je vous épargne la roborative leçon sur la division géométrique du monocorde –, vous saurez, donc, que pour concevoir mathématiquement le ton musical et vous sentir de mèche cabinet secret, il lui est échu de nommer, et il égrène patiemment, détaillant à plaisir folioles, tiges, couleurs et corolles d'icelles, vingt-six figures de style, autant de fleurs aux délicates nervures sonores, Monsieur, dont seize sont des figures de l'harmonie, à savoir fugue réelle, métalepse, hypallage, apocope, *noëma*, analepse, *mimêsis*, anadiplose, *symblêma*, syncope ou synérèse, pléonasme, auxèse, *pathopoeia*, hypotypose, aposiopèse, *anaplokê*, dont six, ensuite, sont de la mélodie, parembole, palillogie, climax, *parrhêsia*, hyperbole, hypobole, et dont quatre, pour clore l'élégante procession, marient la mélodie et l'harmonie, accumulation, *homostikhaonta* – qui est l'autre nom de la progression parallèle, Monsieur – ou *homoiokinéoména* – qui est le mouvement parallèle ou faux-bourdon –, anaphore, fugue imaginaire. Les avez-vous comptés, Monsieur ? Trente-sept solécismes et figures, à quoi s'ajoutent quatre styles, humble, sublime, moyen et mixte, c'est à savoir quarante-et-une entrées, en rangs serrés, dans le grand registre de ce nouvel orgue théorique.

Le maître est artisan, bien plutôt que marchand. Que sert de s'enrichir, quand la seule richesse véritable tient à une tourterelle et à un rameau d'or ? Ses livres, autorisés par les routiniers protecteurs des humanités des Roses, se vendront pour quelques *joachimici*, des écus de Joachim, oui Monsieur, autrement appelés risdales, thalers. Point n'est besoin, j'espère, de vous représenter avec force adjectifs la notoriété que l'auteur et ses ouvrages s'apprêtent à connaître. Comptons, pour solde de toutes veilles, quelques amis dévoués, pontes bienveillants, collègues polis, chalands distraits et autres érudits voyageurs que ravit toujours la vue d'un opus curieux ; peu de lecteurs, donc, tant il est difficile de fonder la rhétorique musicale.

Mais Burmeister se soucie peu de ces hypothétiques gloires terrestres trébuchantes aussitôt que sonnantes qui chez tant d'autres sont le sel d'une vie. Car son plus grand plaisir, dans le vaste atelier à l'odeur tenace où s'affairent l'imprimeur et ses aides, dans ce moulin nouveau où la meule est la presse d'où sort le papier grenu dentelé de noir, son plus grand plaisir est d'observer, jour après jour, le typographe qui, suivant avec application les serpentins et autres menues mouches virevoltantes qu'a dessinés la plume de monsieur l'auteur sur un modeste papier, puise en curieuses petites boîtes maculées d'encre des caractères typographiques de différentes natures, lettres, chiffres, tirets, points, de différentes tailles, l'éloge funèbre du seigneur *magister* Burmeister par le seigneur Docteur Bacmeister ; j'ai lu, lu et relu l'éloge funèbre de Madame Burmeister seconde née Naderheiden par le seigneur Docteur Wasmundt (et sachez que cette petite prose-là, tout particulièrement, est d'une indigence rare, tant il n'est rien à dire sur une simple épouse, sinon qu'elle fut pieuse, eut des parents, des enfants et des proches). Sachez encore, Monsieur, que j'ai lu, lu et relu l'éloge funèbre de la très chère Dorothea Burmeister, décédée à dix-neuf ans, au grand désarroi de son père. Et donc, lorsque j'apprends de la bouche endeuillée de Monsieur le Recteur Thomas Lindeman qui, au dimanche de *Laetare* 1623, célèbre l'envol vers les cieux de la jouvencelle, fille de son très honoré père – lorsque j'apprends, donc, qu'étant enfant, cette âme pure, au moment des repas, récitait à ses parents *les sentences bibliques des livres sacrés, les psaumes de David, les hymnes de D. M. L. et autres pieuses prières* ; que jeune fille, elle récitait, le dimanche et aux jours de fêtes, *les évangiles en entier au repas de midi, et les épîtres en entier au repas du soir* ; qu'elle fut tellement versée dans la lecture de la Bible qu'elle savait proposer *des synopsis des histoires sacrées avec ses propres mots* ; quand je lis tout cela, je crois, je sais, je puis vous assurer qu'il n'en fut point ainsi. Passons sur l'âme pure, la petite carte postale, la jeune fille à la perle (et aussi bien la nôtre, modeste fille de professeur, et non point de marchand, ne porte pas de turban comme chez Monsieur Vermeer) : blanches comme le lys, elles le sont toutes à cet âge-là, ce n'est point d'aujourd'hui – quoique je sois persuadé qu'elle eut l'œil espiègle, noir et brillant d'être si bleu. Mais, Monsieur, pouvez-vous croire, pouvons-nous croire un seul instant à la petite hypotypose de M. Lindeman, à ce petit tableau de sainte famille recomposée auquel, bien avant l'heure, un Greuze de Poméranie apporte la dernière touche, si touchante ? Le voyez-vous en votre esprit, ce tableau ? Imaginez un peu ceci : madame Burmeister née Naderheiden et ses mains pieusement jointes devant sa brune assiette fumante, à sa droite ses garçons Joachim et Christian, pieusement ébouriffés, à sa gauche sa fille Catharina, le rose pieusement vivace aux joues, et en face, avec à sa droite son fils Joachim, son premier Joachim, fils de Joachim et petit-fils de Joachim – et en face, donc, maître Burmeister en Dieu le père, en auguste sénateur siégeant à la sainte table, écoutant doctement, avec hochements de tête d'usage et sourcil aux aguets, sa fille Dorothea qui récite la Bible en langue teutonne. En allemand, oui, en allemand, Monsieur, et c'est petites protestations de modestie éculées – qui arrache, dis-je, à Burmeister, dans sa préface, des confidences sur sa joie et son impatience de faire briller, tinter le rameau d'or, *Musica theorica*, aux yeux et aux oreilles du monde. C'est que désormais, Monsieur, ce rameau doit conduire Burmeister, non dans de quelconques enfers – puisque aussi bien de Sisyphe et du Tartare, il connaît tout –, mais dans les divines contrées des Muses où sonne, et pour toujours, l'ineffable musique des sphères qui accompagne leurs danses. Là-bas, point de rythmes rustiques, point de bourrées et branles rustauds, point de psaumes, point d'hymnes, point de messes, point de culte dominical, point de luthériennes trompettes assaillant des Jéricho papistes promptes à renaître telles les têtes de l'hydre, point de surintendant, point de recteur et corecteur ; non, juste de la musique, Monsieur. Et pour joindre le pays de Musique, le rameau d'or est aussi bien un fil d'Ariane, qui se dévide, se déroule, et vous sort du labyrinthe des servitudes.

Depuis 1609, Burmeister n'écrit plus rien, n'écrira plus rien, ne dira plus rien. Pourquoi écrire ? Pour se rendre immortel ? Mais Monsieur, figurez-vous bien que maître Burmeister est – ou se croit – déjà immortel, depuis qu'en son esprit (certes fatigué par le labeur, et légèrement embrumé, peut-être), le rameau d'or s'est peu à peu mué, cristallisé en lamelles d'or, de ces fameuses lamelles d'or, qui, de toute Antiquité, rendent immortels les sectateurs d'Orphée. Qu'importent à Burmeister les supposées vicissitudes de cette vallée de larmes, lorsqu'il s'absorbe en sa Babel intérieure, y songe et s'abandonne à une rêverie délicieuse ? Souvenez-vous, Monsieur, oui, souvenez-vous, encore et encore, du petit jeune homme en mantelet bleu qui sourit, assoupi, au bord de la Warnow : c'est lui, c'est lui, de toute éternité. Il songe. Et désormais, il le sait, il le sent, *il est enfant de la Terre et du Ciel étoilé, sa lignée est céleste.* Il est un des innombrables fils et émules de la Réforme, oui, mais devenu fils d'Orphée. De la Réforme à Orphée, il n'y a guère qu'un son de moins, me direz-vous, alors que vous attendez peut-être, justement, de courir chez Morphée, lassé que vous êtes de mon petit babil – je plaisante, Monsieur. Mais reprenons car, j'en suis sûr, il vous importe de savoir, enfin, à quoi sert d'être luthérien, quand on est un Burmeister – parce qu'il faut bien que luthérien rime avec autre chose que rien – ; être luthérien, c'est-à-dire rompre avec les fastes des apparences catholiques, se défaire des superstitions, miracles, pèlerinages encoquillés à

Post-scriptum

Aux sources de ce récit se trouvent diverses œuvres anciennes, dont celles écrites, composées ou éditées par Joachim Burmeister, publiées à Rostock entre 1599 et 1609 ; les éloges funèbres prononcés à la mémoire de Dorothea Burmeister, Joachim Burmeister et Dorothea Burmeister née Naderheiden ; les ouvrages de Georg Braun et Frans Hogenberg comportant des cartes de Rostock ; la carte de Wenceslas Hollar ; la chronique consacrée à Rostock par Peter Lindeberg ; sans oublier le registre des immatriculations de l'Université de Rostock.

DEEPAK GUPTA

Copyright © Deepak Gupta 2022

doctors see the end of the visit as the writing of a script.. after having made a snap diagnosis. (Some grab the blood test request form as if it is the holy grail). After all, they know you would be back if the meds did not cure your problem.

Of course, patients simply find other doctors if they are treated badly. Which, of course, does not apply to the state hospital system, where you see a different doctor every time and have no choice in the matter. But most doctors nowadays seem to be wired to get rid of you within your few minutes of allotted time, to move on to the next patient.

This was during the first two years of the illness.

Scornful doctors

I had the experience that one doctor would venture into the field to suggest ME and the next one would laugh in my face and tell me there is no such a disease. (I know at least ten other ME sufferers who can attest to the same scenario having played out in their lives). Imagine how it feels, sitting across from a doctor, feeling so sick you can hardly move, and being laughed at in your face.

This was in the middle nineties when the internet was not yet a click away. Years and years of abusive doctors and medical staff – and all the while, in Europe, America and the East research were moving ahead and answers were being found.

In the UK, already in the nineties, patients with ME would be classified as being disabled, and receive state grants. In that country they recognize the patient's inability and immovability and know how to treat the disease. At that time the average course of the illness was deemed to be 60 months (five years)… for a subset of patients who could regain their health.

In South Africa, to this day, the light has still not reached the medical profession to the degree where doctors know that ME is a disease of the central nervous system, as classified by WHO (World Health Organization). Even neurologists do not know this – really.

No wonder then, that most patients with ME (and I have met quite a few) eventually turn their backs on the medical fraternity and start looking for answers in the alternative or complementary fields. Some of this is quackery and some even possibly dangerous. The sad news is that people who are so ill that they can hardly stand upright for a few hours per day, have to contend with this bewildering wilderness of unhelpful medical staff, disbelieving friends, and very helpful but often questionable alternative methodologies…

It may sound exaggerated, but this is a depiction of the very real truth as experienced by hundreds of thousands of people out there. Global incidence of ME is estimated at between 1 and 2 percent of the world's population: millions of people.

Personally, I eventually, around the third year of finding no answers and little relief, ventured into the alternative medicine field – and found value in quite a few places, but with careful prior research. I am not the kind of person who would willy nilly leap into the unknown – even though I was more than desperate at times.

And this desperation was not just to stay alive… but to FEEL alive. I know there are millions of people who can relate to this, some with fatal diseases. Some have to cope with being bound to a bed, with tubes and machines and equipment. Thank God, I do not have experience of this.

Nevertheless, I have been left with feeling less than alive – the feeling that I am carrying within me the numbing sensation of being more dead than alive. Hmm, I can hear some think this is a psychological nut case. I am neither neurotic nor psychotic nor schizophrenic… but am a person who had to battle the fatigue in my muscles and the concomitant neurological disadvantages as well as the polyneuropathy I have been left with… not to mention the numerous food allergies and intolerances which remain more than a passing complication, with pathetically little support coming from medical sources.

Psychological impact

Over the years, I have wondered about the psychological impact of this off-handed (in most cases) and in some instances hostile - treatment received at the hands of medical staff. Are doctors and nursing staff in their training ever given the insight that their attitudes, their words and actions, play a role in how a patient perceives his illness, even his life? And how this perception affects the outcome of his disease? From my own experience this did not seem to be the case.

One example: one day at the Steve Biko hospital, while the lambs were waiting for the doctors to complete their rounds and come to the clinic, the nurses offered us tea.. can you believe it. Just this simple gesture of kindness lifted the mood perceptibly. It made the waiting more bearable, and the people feel more human.

I have had so many different diagnoses it now makes me laugh. I was not laughing at the time! It is small wonder that those with the most modern syndromes (Fibromyalgia, Restless Legs Syndrome, and ME – now referred to as Chronic Fatigue Syndrome) give up on the medical fraternity at some point and turn their backs on what is most likely nothing other than a drawn-out bad experience, not culminating in answers, treatment or improvement.

I have been told that I had an incurable disease, for which there was no treatment. The same person told me I would end up in a care facility, immobile and unable to feed myself. Another visit to hospital left me with being told that they will have to amputate both my feet. Really? At age 51 I started running again... and last year was awarded provincial colors in cross country running. Imagine how I felt standing in the starting line at the SA national championships!

However, I am not highlighting here anything other than the fact that medical staff makes many statements to patients in an off-handed way –

not thinking about the damage they are causing to the person's overall outlook on life… if you are told you will lose both your feet… how would it make you feel? Happy? Hopeful? Luckily I disregarded most of what I was told, since by this time I was emotionally desensitized – reflecting on an emotional level my body's state of being. And seriously (and possibly incurably) distrustful of medical doctors!

I suspect that most patients with inexplicable symptoms, who are in excruciating chronic pain, eventually become emotionally distant as a coping mechanism for dealing with the pain. If you feel the physical pain with your emotions, it becomes that much worse. And yet, sometimes you cannot do otherwise. Pain eventually tramples down enthusiasm as time goes by.

Some days were downright dreadful. Particularly those following on a night of little sleep… When you had to drag yourself out of bed, force yourself to face the day, and felt as if you were pulling a load behind you (or in you) like Robert de Niro going up the waterfall in The Mission. When the cells in your body seemed to be shouting in protest, and your brain had to try and shout louder to have its commands heard. When your muscles fail to comply, now *that* is the place where the rubber hits the road.

And then the stark realization that you are having to do battle against the very healthcare system that is supposed to help you – adding in spades to the load of being physically ill.

What is ME?

The WHO (World Health Organization) classified ME as a disease of the central nervous system. Research has shown that the brain stem can be involved, due to reduced blood flow (hypoperfusion).

The CDC (Centers for Disease Control) criteria for a diagnosis of ME are:

1) Clinically evaluated persistent or relapsing fatigue
2) Concurrent occurrence of at least four of the following symptoms:

impairment in short-term memory
sore throat
tender lymph nodes
muscle pain
headaches
unrefreshing sleep
multi-joint pain
tiredness after exertion lasting more than 24 hours

My own, short definition is total system shutdown. And last year, in 2019, Jarred Younger Ph.D., at the Open Medicine Foundation conference, described it as "brain inflammation that attacks the muscles". Of all the definitions and descriptions I have heard, this is the most direct and best.

Chapter Three

Finding the cause

The quest for the cause of one's disease can become a goal in itself. This is almost inevitable in the early stages of a disease. Yet it can waylay your recovery if taken to the extreme. However, I have never met anyone who could blithely accept the symptoms without wanting to find the cause. It seems to me an action as natural as breathing. Also, I am convinced that part of learning to deal with the symptoms is to discover its origin. Therefore, the search for the cause is inevitable.

I have known people who advised me not to give my illness a name. "Do not give it a name – you are bringing illness onto yourself", I was told.

This, according to them, would be akin to giving Satan the authority to afflict me (as if it was not happening already). Yet in my own experience and from talking to many people with a variety of chronic conditions, I gained the impression that identifying the illness, and the cause thereof, is not just necessary from a treatment point of view, but it is an empowering step seen from a psychological perspective.

Even if one shuns the idea of consulting a doctor - or is simply not able to do so - and holds to fighting the disease without medical intervention, this remains true. Knowing what you are dealing with, what you are facing, gives you the power to make decisions about how to go about fighting it – both psychologically and in terms of treatment, lifestyle changes, dietary changes, and the like.

(I feel the need to stress here that I felt too weak to fight for many a year, and that I was basically just coping, and not moving forward. I can say this about the first ten years at the very least.)

Since this is not a book about ME per se, I am sharing only limited information about symptoms, treatment or changes. I do want to point out that multi-factorial syndromes are a bit beyond the norm of well-known disease conditions with established treatment paradigms.

Still today, well into the 22nd century, in South Africa confusion reigns about ME and very little progress has been made with educating doctors as well as the public at large. I can quite understand this conundrum... I once posed the question to a doctor about where they learn the latest about disease and treatment. The answer was in medical journals.

Money Talks

At that time I was the managing editor of a medical journal. When I proposed an article on this topic to the publisher, the question was: who would advertise next to the article? Of course, there was no known drug treatment for it – ergo – no article, no education of doctors. Of course, were there a drug company that had developed a drug that they needed to sell – education would have been a given. This is where patients are cast into the doldrums and left to fend for themselves.

Is it surprising that people eventually come to the conclusion that money talks – also in the medical field? If your disease condition means money could be made out of it by drug companies or medical equipment suppliers, you would be borne on the wave of treatment quite happily – for as long as your medical aid continues to pay the bills, of course. It is

Into the picture of confusion, and adding to it in a more than minute way, stepped the media with its "yuppie flu" description, which in no time at all became the accepted cultural narrative of our time – making a mockery of a serious, debilitating condition and adding its own stigma - which, on its own, is a battle to behold. Stripping an illness of its validity means the sick person is regarded as not being sick, and many a scurrilous explanation is put forward for their illness. I am rather certain that no-one this ill would want to be sick or stay sick, therefore treating them as if they are not, makes getting well that much harder for the powerless patient.

Some diseases can be a singular problem – but a disease like ME is a plural disease (syndrome) with a complex series of symptoms, problems and pain platforms to traverse.

In many cases, CFS is like a build-up of infections, mostly viral, in which the immune system eventually says enough is enough and its responses cannot meet the load anymore. On one occasion I saw this quite clearly (and this was about seven years after the acute phase of the illness) when a naturopathic doctor tested my blood every week to determine what was happening and why my sinus infection was not clearing up. It took seven weeks for my body to start making white blood cells to fight the infection, a response which should have taken less than 24 hours.

Clinical or reactive depression?

The number of times I have been told I suffer from depression, well, many a time this came from a doctor's lips. Yes, of course you will become depressed at some stage. I would like to see a person with chronic fatigue and chronic pain, who do not (eventually) feel depressed. However, this is reactive depression, a result of being sick and not finding the cause, or treatment, or being given any hope – this is not genetic or clinical or anything other than the result of the circumstances!

I told a doctor who offered me Prozac that I would flush it down the toilet. (This was after she denigrated my physical symptoms and became nasty). Despite my hopeless situation, my mental strength was way beyond what she could have imagined, even though I looked, and sounded, depressed. I do know that neurological symptoms other than depression are being treated with anti-depressants and even anti-epileptic medication. I have over time formulated my own non-medical way of dealing with this, since I do not believe one needs psychotropic drugs unless you are clinically depressed or have clinically proven epilepsy.

This is my way of looking at it, therefore do not take this as being instructive in terms of your own situation. Ultimately each person makes his own choices and taking into account everything you have been told, have read, researched and experienced, you will find your own way. If this means medical drug treatment, so be it. For me, it was not.

Chapter Four

Sleeping in the arms of ME's "disaster of symptoms"

With acknowledgment to Prof Ron Tompkins of Harvard Medical School who coined this phrase.

Right now in 2020, the dizziness I have come to know, is worse than ever. Sometimes the lightheaded feeling is so bad that I need to sit down. I cannot turn my head for fear of turning the earth's axis on itself. And while running, well, it becomes worse. For several hours after running it remains in pumped-up state, and then returns to "normal". Why is it getting worse? No idea.

"I think you suffer from orthostatic hypotension" my doctor said during one visit in 1997. She went on to explain that this means my blood pressure changes dramatically when I change position, such as sitting up after lying down. She took my blood pressure while lying back, sitting up, standing up, squatting on my haunches and standing up again – and was proven to be correct. Especially the latter caused a big fall in blood pressure. To this day, despite all my running and exercising, going down on my haunches is something I avoid. I also take care not to get up too fast.

Ever heard of POTS? It seems that there is a correlation with ME/CFS. Postural Orthostatic Tachycardia Syndrome means changes in blood pressure put so much pressure on the heart that the patient gets tachycardia (heart palpitations). In my world, palpitations are so common that I usually take note of it in passing. Of course, mine is probably mild compared with other people.

And as for dizziness, one fine day while running a cross country race I was so dizzy I felt that if I should close my eyes I would most certainly faint. So, the answer to that was – do not think of your dizziness. Think of your running. Keep going. And thus I reached the finish line, dizzy or not!

Have I tried to find an answer to this dizziness? Or course I have. But apart from taking my blood pressure and listening to my heart no-one seems to think that dizziness as a symptom needs to be taken seriously.

Jogging along with the dizziness, sometimes in pace but often way ahead, is tinnitus: ringing in the ears. Mine has been on the left side since (I think) 1971. Over the years it intensified. Now, while I am deemed healthy, this problem persists. When I lie down the ringing becomes more persistent. I try not to move my head because it is intrusive. I have had my ears tested. Nothing wrong with my hearing.

In trying to address this I have found that it requires a very costly in-ear aid which emits white noise that dampens the ringing sound. Might I mention that research into tinnitus shows that it comes from the brain, not the ears *per se*. Sitting in a noisy restaurant is the one place where tinnitus does not bother you. Sitting in a quiet library – the ringing rolls around my head like waves coming in to shore.

I still, after 23 years, have no answer to these two problems. They are as persistent as my insomnia. Did I mention sleep in the title of this chapter? Sleeping is as elusive as Prince Charming...

When I was in the acute phase of ME/CFS, I had hypersomnia. I slept and slept and woke up in a daze feeling as if I had not slept for days. Thus, the unrefreshing sleep CFS bestows upon you. Following in its wake, sleeping problems. Insomnia – mine is not the "cannot get to sleep" variety. No, I reach the point during the early evening where I am so tired, I just cannot stay awake. Then I wake up (usually abruptly) somewhere around midnight and start staring at the ceiling.

I never get more than four hours of sleep in this first-pass nightly ritual. The second pass could be either lying awake for hours, or when I am lucky I might be awake for a short space of time and fall asleep again. More often, though, I battle on, waiting expectantly for the birds to start singing around 4 am when I give up trying to fall asleep and get up to start the day.

One doctor who attempted to help me solve this problem prescribed an anti-epileptic. Oh what a night! Soon after drinking the tablet, I walked into the doorway. I became disoriented and woozy. BUT!!! My eye muscles went into spasm and I could not close my eyes. I sat on my bed, bug-eyed and awake, until morning came. Needless to say I called the doc and he was stumped. "Never heard of this happening" he apologetically said. I had such a good rapport with this doctor that I felt sorry for him!

Anti-seizure medication, anti-anxiety meds, antidepressants, sleeping tablets. All of these had such serious side effects that I (by my own choice) avoid them altogether. Just recently my doctor suggested taking melatonin (the hormonal precursor used by the brain to slow you down to sleep).

This also did not help me. I would sleep for three hours and wake up. After a period of being wide awake I would enter a field of not being awake, but not being asleep, either. Lying in this state, listening to car doors slamming, the neighbor's bedroom gymnastics, while waiting for the birds…. No thanks. I will battle on and take my sleep where I can find it.

Long term sleep deprivation in itself has more consequences than the obvious daytime drowsiness and cognitive slowing down. Some of the effects are irritability, fatigue, clumsiness (oh yes), forgetfulness, difficulty with concentration, carbohydrate cravings, moodiness, depression, and a weakened immune system.

Talking about cognitive function – I have a long history of hypoglycemia, which in itself causes rather unpleasant symptoms, which are blithely ignored by all and sundry: dizziness, blurred vision, feeling shaky (my hands actually shake), inability to concentrate... these could lead to more serious symptoms including seizures and loss of consciousness. This actually sounds like sleep deprivation.. so putting the two together makes for fun times.

I have yet to find someone who takes you seriously when you say your blood sugar is low. One morning I almost fainted in a hospital reception area, and when I took the lady by the arm and said I felt as if I was about to faint, she just ignored me.

Experience taught me to keep my blood sugar level up by eating carbs. I cannot take sugar. Even a glass of fruit juice (or a fruit salad) puts my body out of commission. Thus those who know me see me eating peanuts and chips at intervals, between small meals.

When I started running, this was of concern to me. How and how much and what to eat became a mission. I completed a sports nutrition course but this did not, of course take into consideration that I am allergic to milk and intolerant to wheat, soya and so on. It has been a rollercoaster trial and error experience, sorting out what I should be doing diet-wise. But I managed to find answers that work for me.

Is low blood sugar connected to candida overgrowth? I am not sure. But although the hypothesis in 1997 was that I had severe candida problems, tests showed it to be insignificant. I was however, treated for gut inflammation and leaky gut, which I most certainly had.

Now, years later, OMF research has shown that inflammatory response changes the brain functions in ME/CFS patients, and induces the sickness response. Once in a hypersensitive state a patient can move in and out of the state of being severely ill even more than once a day, explains Dr. Jarred Younger (Ph.D.). This is why a two-minute walk can make a patient feel sick, he explains. His research also showed a high incidence of lactate in the brains of ME/CFS patients – indicative of neuroinflammation.

These patients experience "hot brain" symptoms- and the spots where the brain's temperature is elevated, coincides with the areas of increased lactate. Based on this research alone – let alone all the other findings that have accumulated over the years – I cannot help but want to throw my hands in the air in despair. Why are patients still being treated as if they are dreaming up symptoms???!

List of symptoms/problems I have experienced:

1. Low blood pressure
2. Orthostatic hypotension
3. Immune dysfunction
4. Leaky gut syndrome
5. Candida
6. Myalgia
7. Muscle spasms
8. Sciatica
9. Dizziness
10. Tinnitus
11. POTS
12. Distal polyneuralgia/neuropathy
13. Occipital neuralgia and neuritis
14. Cognitive dysfunction
15. Allergies: food, airborne and others
16. Food intolerances

It is important to remember that homeopathic treatment is systemic and therefore is a far cry from taking a substance that will alleviate (or deaden) the pain. I have had the benefit of consulting doctors who started in the medical field and extended their expertise into homeopathy. Straddling both disciplines is, of course, beneficial to patients. Naturopathic help also made a huge impact and might I say my first step back to health was dietary adjustments. Never again will I think of food as just pleasure. I see food as medicine and prefer to right nutritional imbalances with food rather than supplements although I do use them when I deem it necessary.

Doing this takes extensive research and dedication. Being responsible about it is of course, essential. I know someone who went on a forty-day fast to kill the Candida in her system. However, after this she had major difficulty with gaining enough weight to return to normal.

Taking your health into your own hands

Perhaps the mind shift comes when you start thinking of yourself as your own physician. How many times have you heard that you know your own body best? I think this eventually becomes true for people who battle long-term chronic disease conditions. I reached the point where I was so aware of nuances and incremental changes that I became competent at nutritional, herbal and supplemental modalities.

Not every person would go to the lengths I have gone to in studying and researching different methods and treatments. But with the ready availability of the internet now, medical information, as well as alternatives, are at hand 24/7. Therefore, people can arm themselves with verifiable information and knowledge. There is also an inherent danger. It would be wise to bear in mind that websites are oftentimes nothing more than online shops used to sell products, while they pose as information sources. Go for medical research sites and test the information put forth against this.

Remember that there is no such thing as a panacea – a single answer for every conceivable problem, or a "magic bullet". Quacks usually try to convince you that no matter what your symptoms, their product will heal or cure you. This is not true. Furthermore, if you add something to your body, even nutritional supplements, you have to bear in mind that something else in the metabolic cascade will be affected.

Chronic pain sufferers are teetering on the brink of hopelessness, facing despair, and can thus easily fall into the trap of believing the next "wonder painkiller" will end all their suffering. This makes them easy targets. Norman Cousins pointed out (so long ago…) that 90% of pain is self-limiting. This means the pain is confined within certain parameters of both time and severity. Now if only one could have the heads up when the pain strikes, then so much spent on medical costs could be avoided, not so?

Carefully consider the consequences

For instance, if you take potassium supplements, your kidneys will be given an extra task and your mineral balance, including that of magnesium and sodium, will be affected. It is always best to start taking supplements only after tests have confirmed that you do have a deficiency. Of course, this is almost impossible (tests being expensive), but taking supplements only after very careful consideration should be the norm: what supplements/prescription medications are you taking already, read up how the supplement could possibly interact (or be blocked) by the food you ingest. Spinach, for eg, blocks the uptake of iron.

The most important reality of all is that the body is an integrated whole. Medicine, due to how it developed, has had to rely on the reductive model because our Western medical knowledge was gained from death – after all, our centuries-old knowledge of the human body is based on dissecting cadavers, quite understandably. This is the reductionist way of looking at the functions of the systems of the body in Western medicine, and unfortunately, very often, in isolation.

This is what I have against specialists (sorry) but you are being naïve in thinking a neurologist would be interested in an endocrine problem… even though the body is, or should function, like an integrated whole. A specialist looks only at his area of specialty and therefore, if your symptoms fall outside of his field, he will send you on your way without a backward glance.

Of course in recent years, magnetic resonance imaging and other functional imaging techniques have made studies of the body's functions possible and have changed this way of thinking of the body as a mechanical composition of different systems, to some degree. It has however not made a major impact on the medical fraternity as a whole.

Thinking of the body as a collection of separate systems, for example, the respiratory system, the nervous system, and the digestive system, (among others) leads to us thinking that anything relating to the digestive system resides there alone. But what about the fact that the immune system creates its ammunition in the digestive tract – and is in fact reliant on the nutrients coming down from above, to be able to do so? Ignoring this means that we do not take care to arm the immune system with the ammunition we, as humans can give it, by eating correctly.

Body intelligence

Take for instance what happens when you cut your finger. The skin, muscles and capillary system are immediately involved. As are the blood and the immune cells which rush to the site with alacrity… and the correct amount of whatever is needed is released. Much more than the various systems are involved here. The body's innate intelligence responds to each and every nuance that takes place in its 50 trillion cells. Deepak Chopra calls it "The delicate web of intelligence that binds the body together".

Some breakthrough thoughts that I eventually came to embrace, are among others, that each person has been given the responsibility for his/her own body. Lifestyle diseases are caused by human choices – treated by doctors and competently financed by collective funding mechanisms. In recent years the media has gone to great lengths to educate the masses about preventative lifestyle choices. Yet, people still rely on bypass surgery and many other medical techniques and pharmaceutical substances to fix the dis-ease they have themselves created.

Type 2 diabetes is perhaps the best example of the masses having the information at their fingertips, yet every year sees more millions around the globe added to the mountain of people who have to rely on medication to maintain their health while living with a degenerative disease and eventually succumbing to its raging ravages.

Knowledge alone is not enough. Change is needed – it can be controlled and arrested, and of course it can be prevented, yet the burden as regards diabetes-related problems is among the highest of burden of disease.

It took me a while to realize that doctors are not there to heal patients: but to treat their symptoms. Lifestyle diseases, as a case in point, are incurable and can only be treated with an armory of drugs and surgery. How many patients walk away – healed?

And on to the body as an intelligent system. Why do we think of the foot as being something apart/separated from the heart? The two are linked in more ways than the obvious. Every cell is in communication with every other cell… and this intelligence is the elusive life force medical science cannot yet find a description for. Chopra, when writing about the scientific breakthrough of the findings of neuropeptides, says "life itself is intelligence riding everywhere on chemicals… and intelligence is free to go where it likes, even where molecules cannot." Neuropeptides have been found everywhere in the body, not just in the brain.

We have it within ourselves to fight disease – consider how Norman Cousins when receiving the prognosis – that he would surely die – used his own intellect and with the assistance of his doctor, fought back and won the fight. He writes in his book "The Anatomy of Illness" (Bantam Books 1979) "studies show that up to 90% of patients who reach out for medical help are suffering from self-limiting disorders well within the range of the body's own healing powers."

Patterns

Us humans instinctively respond to input the brain can distinguish as a recognizable pattern. Until the chaos settles into a pattern, it is just a chaos of intelligent information. The brain works with pattern recognition. What is reading other than pre-learned recognition of symbolic patterns on a page? Reasoning too is dependent upon recognizing a pattern and then responding to it – also scientific reasoning, which includes the way doctors are taught to reach a diagnosis.

Driving a car is a set of learned patterns, as is following a recipe or making a braid in your hair or typing something in Microsoft Word. In the case of the car, if the pattern is not followed, mechanical damage would result, as would the recipe result in an inedible mess if you get one of the crucial steps wrong.

In the same way, medical doctors treat patients according to recognized patterns; sets of symptoms presenting in a certain way indicate a certain condition. Medical students are taught the scientific paradigm of recognizable patterns. Something needs to be identified as a pattern and then treated in a set paradigm. Take for instance the booklet handed to a child with asthma. Coded in red, orange and green... each set of symptoms described and prescribed for in a predetermined way. This in itself is not negative. It is quite sensible. Yet it is also limiting since it pertains only to the known, easily treatable disease conditions.

However, there is much beyond the pattern that is excluded merely because the pattern has become the norm. This is why doctors find it so difficult to treat patients presenting with ME/CFS – because it defies every pattern identified until now… and by the way, it is not the only disease condition to do so. But by and large doctors seem stumped when they cannot make it fit into one of the boxes they learned about in med school. In most instances I have experienced, doctors find it close to impossible to rise above their professional indoctrination.

Chapter Six

People's reactions

When you fall ill, you respond in a uniquely personal way. Initially you are not aware of how other people respond to you in turn. But in due time, you are almost slapped in the face by other people's reactions. Finding answers to why you are ill… I found in general, few people could deal with not knowing what was wrong, why you were sick and could not seem to get better… they needed a name, a diagnosis, a cause, to relate to you. I often felt like telling them that their responses were putting pressure on me that I did not need adding to the load I was already carrying!

I sometimes wondered how different people's reactions would have been if I had answered "Cancer" to their questions. Would they have showered me with love/care/affection/pity? Just because they happened to know about the disease?

People lost interest pretty soon when they had asked me more than once what was wrong and could not be given a pat answer. By the third time they had stopped asking. And I stopped talking about it. Not feeling well, having pain, possible causes, possible treatments, after all, were topics interesting only to the one involved.

On the other hand, I often wished people would let it go because some persisted in telling you what you should do (even though they had less than a clue about your situation). I had many people, upon hearing about the pain in my legs, rushing in with advice about taking magnesium. Well now, firstly I was not experiencing cramps (which magnesium is indicated

Being alone is not necessarily the only thing that makes you feel isolated. You could be with a group of people, or some people I know, with a partner, who, failing to understand or be supportive, make you feel as isolated as the one who is physically alone all (or most) of the time. It almost feels like being in a bubble from which you are trying – but failing – to reach out to others in a normal way.

The feeling of isolation became stronger each time after I had interaction with a doctor or some person who failed to understand. Ultimately you start feeling as if you have to defend yourself against people who are supposed to help you... and feeling defensive leads to feeling isolated on a plane where no-one else can reach out and touch you.

I can just imagine what it must feel like spending months in a hospital bed – phew. That must really isolate a patient and make him feel inhuman.

I started working as a freelance writer and managed to work from home, which made it possible for me to earn an income. It also served to reinforce my isolation – sometimes weeks went by without me speaking to even one person outside my home. The internet, too, thankfully, was an enabler that allowed me to, despite my situation, put through large volumes of work without having to leave my home. Yet this, too, exacerbated my isolation.

Chapter Seven

The meaning of life = falling down fatigued

To most people, at some or other time in their lives, they reach the point of thinking of and seeking answers, to the question of what their lives really mean.

Viktor Frankl even wrote his famous book Man's Search for Meaning (1946), postulating answers to this question. Tracing the horrifying events in the concentration camps during WWII, and describing how some people, if they find, and can hold on to, the idea that their life has a certain meaning, will overcome almost impossible obstacles in the quest to remain alive, he found. In this, Nietzsche's statement was proved to be correct, when he said "he who has a why to live can bear almost any how".

I have been thinking about this incessantly over the years. I have not found this elusive meaning in my life. Not in the esoteric, airy-fairy way in which I can ever describe the meaning of my life as anything other than staying alive. No major, all-consuming goal, no quest for a cause, or anything other than helping my child grow up and staying on my feet from one day to the next.

Since I was working as a missionary at the time of becoming ill, I did not doubt the (higher) meaning of my life just before falling down fatigued, unable to move or think, or question. In those dark days I did not question the meaning of what was happening to me. Engulfing pain has the distinct ability to drown out other thoughts, whatever they may be. Gordon Allport pointed out that at every moment man's mind is directed by some intention. Sure. But when in pain, your intention fixes its focus on the pain, how to deal with it, or more pressingly, how to get rid of it. It took me years to get over this need to rid myself of physical pain and to rather focus on dealing with what I could not change in the best possible way.

Frankl pointed out the difficulty in this: "If we make health our main concern we have fallen ill – we have become hypochondriacs." I understand this statement – in the context of healthy people fixating on their health. For a person with chronic pain though, it becomes almost impossible to think of anything else. I read somewhere that someone talked about "the pain that drowns out faith" and found this resonating with where I was at. My pain drowned out everything, including my personality.

Having moved from wanting to be rid of the pain, to find mechanisms to cope with it was a meaningful step. This did not happen overnight. Being in constant wracking pain is like being on a flat-bottom boat being cast this way and that by waves all around, and not being able to steer the boat yourself. Even at this moment my body is in pain. But I became adept at pushing it down into my subconscious and getting on with my day despite the discomfort it caused me. There are still those days when pain is overwhelming in its intensity. Those grit-your-teeth and grin-and-bear-it days. I have experienced countless days like this.

I made a decision years ago to tackle the pain alone, with only supplements and natural treatments (and my own intelligence) and therefore painkillers did not feature except in really desperate moments. Even when I do use pain killers, I do not exceed the bottom-line 500mg paracetamol dosage.

I have seen too much in terms of my own body's response to medication, which was everything but predictable and in some instances downright inexplicable. For example, a medication that should have calmed down the brain's electrical workings, did the opposite and I spent an entire night sitting upright in my bed, with my eye muscles in spasm!

Back to the meaning in all of this... what could be the meaning of overriding pain? There are millions of people asking this question every day. Perhaps the pain is pointing you to a place within yourself, which only you and your Maker can access. Maybe this is the very place to meet Him - and your real self, too.

I see many driven people – driven by their careers, and even more people driven by their children's lives. They shape their lives, and their selves, around something outside themselves. Perhaps that's not all bad, but in the process, do they lose their own selves? Could this be the meaning of pain in your body—***to get you in contact with yourself*** on a level you would never have attained otherwise? I am not saying this is the answer... I am contemplating this and have been doing so for years.

I am sure this is not so for everyone landing in a pit of pain. My own life was not lead in reckless abandon – I was after all, working as a missionary at the time of becoming ill. Yet I was also denying myself and my own needs and psychological welfare *in toto*. This was self-destructive, but at the time, I saw no other way of applying my calling to serve God. May I add that I was alone and had no support from the people who sent me to another country with only the laying on of hands and a prayer.

I can now see, looking back, just how naïvely I put myself in the hands of others who, in the name of Jesus, abused my unconditional willingness to serve. I did not know it at the time, but some other people had agendas that were altogether dishonorable – and they made me play an unwitting part in their schemes!

Finding meaning in a situation like that? Well, I have never blamed anyone for the decisions I made. What they did certainly had an impact on my life. But, having moved on after discovering the treachery and dishonesty of the people I had trusted, I still hold myself accountable for my own decisions – including the wrong ones!

Pain itself – chronic pain that is, has no inherent meaning. Acute pain, on the other hand, tells you that something needs urgent attention. But throbbing, dull pain that refuses to shift, perhaps its purpose has existential meaning only?

Albert Einstein said "The man who regards his life as meaningless is not merely unhappy but hardly fit for life". I wonder though, how many people stop and consider the meaning of their lives on a level deeper than the everyday getting-through-life situations? It did, after all take me some time…

It is easy to accept that God placed you on the earth and that in itself has meaning. But… finding the value in pain and disability?

Finding meaning in having a chronic disease is not easy. It is not the same for every sick person either. Some days being in pain takes on the lofty existential meaning I am talking about – and other days, it is just merely a physical pain that irks me as well as hurts my muscles. Remember too that pain most often leads to debilitating difficulties. Going up a flight of stairs… the pain exacerbates the difficulty with which the task has to be completed.

Many centuries ago Hippocrates, whom we regard as the father of medicine, said: "A wise man should consider that health is the greatest of human blessings and how by his own thoughts to derive benefit from his illness". The same vaunted philosopher also said: "to do nothing is also a good remedy." Therefore as I am illustrating here, meaning is to be found in adversity. In the case of physical illness we have been trained to seek the help of others. Is this not preventing us from finding meaning in our situation?

Frankl suggested that what we regard as midlife crisis, is likely to be a point where people (men and women) start thinking about the meaning of their lives – and he calls it an existential crisis, a feeling of futility, and the overall realization that you are existentially frustrated. Many people then make changes to their lives, yet the change they seek is to find meaning for themselves, not in changing the surroundings.

Do you wish to die, or just to stop living?

As I have mentioned, my quest for health was not an easy one. Many a day I opened my eyes, with the thought that I had to get up and get through one more day… and with nothing to look forward to in this process but difficulty in walking, pain, brain fog, and who knows what else.. since symptoms and infections, would come and go with no discernible pattern, no warning and no breathing space.

In 2006 (nine years after my first encounter with ME/CFS) I went to the zoo one night at the end of March. The next day I had a full-on lung infection and coughed like a 40 Texan-plain smoker. That year bronchitis was followed by pneumonia and pleurisy which was followed by another bout of bronchitis – and I coughed all the way into September when I left for Italy. This was no joke – medication could not shift the recurrent infections and I was helpless in the face of the constant wracking cough –

and wondering how people with emphysema could fail to stop their smoking habit (those who keep on smoking, of course).

Helpless and without a reason to live – I wanted to die. I really did. I prayed to God to let me die. I did not die. But I also did not want to live. I did not have the driving will to stay alive that Viktor Frankl talks about in Man's Search for Meaning. Really. I had nothing to look forward to. Despite my heartfelt wishes to be dead, I forced myself to get up and do everything I could to get through the day, meaningful or not.

Getting through one day at a time became my motto, and it still is. I could no longer plan things weeks in advance since I had no way of knowing whether I would be able to stay on my feet on a certain day. I also had to learn to stop feeling guilty about the things I could not do. Friends most certainly started seeing me as unreliable since I sometimes had to cancel planned things just hours before. This was a contrary thing for me. I had to learn to distance myself from feelings like guilt and incompetence.

In fact, I had to learn to distance myself from a large number of my emotions. Sadness, unhappiness, guilt, and so on. On the one hand you have to learn to acknowledge your emotions, and on the other hand, not to be driven by them. These are some of the things I learned this courtesy of the illness – but it was not as if I got these abilities for free. It was acquired at great cost.

First of all, apathy is the result. Getting from apathy back to being in touch with, and allowing yourself to experience emotions, is a lesson in itself, one which takes months, even years to learn.

Anyway, there is a difference between wanting to die, and wanting to stop living. Many people who experience excruciating pain wish to be free of pain – to sink into total oblivion and not feel anything anymore. They are in fact hoping to stop living because living has become unbearably painful for them. Wanting to die might signify a person's understanding that life on the other side of physical being could be better than what he

Being limited to crawling on all fours will bring home to you just how much you had always taken for granted. I have read of people living like this for years, thankfully my own initial period of acute illness lasted a few months, after which I slowly – always excruciatingly slowly – managed to get around and at least regain some modicum of being human.

Honestly, I did not care. I had no way of caring what I looked like when at the time, I would wake in blackness, not knowing what day of the week or time of day it was. Who cared? I had no way of connecting with myself, never mind connecting with others. I felt disconnected, adrift, and alone. Alone with nothing but my thoughts and my shattered body.

Left in this state, one of the many questions that form in one's mind is assuredly the question of what is real… and what is not. Is life real? Is health real? Am I real? Is God real? What is reality, after all? I could not answer any of these questions in a way that would satisfy anyone, most of all myself. Right now, I still ponder these questions, and their answers. And perhaps have added some knowledge, wisdom and experience to the contemplation of the answers.

Is life real? Well, perhaps in the measure in which you are consciously aware of it. That's what we generally refer to as being alive. Yet, most people, whilst being alive, having life in their bodies, are not consciously tuned in, thinking of being alive and what it means. This question of course, is a relevant one to any person with a life-threatening illness. They are the ones who ponder this. Maybe because they are forced into doing so - and cannot escape doing it. Others, for whom the bells are not tolling, live their lives as if its value is interchangeable.

Some years later, being avidly interested in varying aspects of things relating to life, I came across in reading about quantum physics, the theory of Schrödinger's cat. This notion that something only becomes real when you observe it to be, makes a mockery of those who see reality in concrete things. That's all of us. His theory that the molecules that make up the table on which my laptop now rests, only becomes reality when I perceive the table and the laptop, while the molecules could in a parallel universe have been something else if they had been perceived there first, was something which caused me much thought.

How about emotions, then? How real are the fleeting emotions that are caused by our senses bringing about biochemical changes in the brain and making us feel and react in a certain way? Are we building everything on shifting sand? It depends on your spiritual belief, how this notion of concrete or shifting reality, will affect you.

The fight to feel normal

In those early days, I used to look at people while they were talking, trying to follow their conversations. I found myself looking at their lips moving and wondering what they were saying. Many times I would silently wonder if they were on to me – whether they could see, could discern that I was struggling to follow. Later on I started wondering whether they could judge that I was not normal and that they would call me out for pretending. To this day I am cognizant of not feeling normal, even though I may seem to be. More than twenty years since that dark dawn descended on me – and still I am not certain what normal is. I am furthermore aware that my emotional responses are different from that of other people. Abnormal – maybe not – but certainly different.

Perhaps I have become a little touchy, since I perceive people to be treating me as if I am stupid – because I know I am not. Just as I am but all too aware that I am not as sharp as I used to be. I remember playing in the big leagues – working round the clock and having the ultimate sense of achievement of success of a job well done. I can still do it. I believe I still can. But my body denies me the ability to go for 20 hours non-stop for weeks at a time, even though my brain goes round the clock at a pace belying my body's grinding refusal to cooperate. My brain refuses to let go.

Let go... now there are two weighty words to contemplate.

Since that early dawn I have had to let go of much. The things I used to do, the things I used to love doing, like singing, playing music, dancing –

became unreachable and undoable. I could not stay upright, never mind stand and sing for hours at a time. I had become a motionless onlooker, unable to do what I took for granted and what I loved.

I will never again live mindlessly, not considering my actions in real-time.

Chapter Nine

The battle with pain

There will be many reading this that will immediately relate to this description.

Sitting in a meeting, the pain threatens to rise to the surface. On occasion it does, and a grimace involuntarily passes across my face. I always cling to the hope that other people do not notice. I am writing this in the present tense because it has now been with me from the very beginning and still wraps me in a fog of pain at times. Thankfully, it is not severe all the time, it comes and goes. In the early days it was so bad it almost smothered me like an Anaconda wrapping itself around my entire being. Guess what, when pain overrides every other sensation in your body, little is left of your mental resources.

The wide divide

Over time I became aware of the wide divide between doing things unconsciously and having to think about something before doing it – such as moving my legs, or arms. That first morning when no part of my body wanted to move, despite my brain saying it was time to get up, was a wake-up call, all right. Most people (probably all people) never spare a thought about HOW to get their legs to move, or which movement has to precede another to get the body in an upright position. Lying in that bed, and wanting to move, but not being able to, was, apart from the physical impossibility, also nearly impossible to explain to others.

Thus, it set me on the path to discover more about the brain – or rather, the mind. The Oxford Dictionary defines mind as "the element of a person that enables them to be aware of the world and their experiences, to think, to feel; the faculty of consciousness and thoughts." The brain is not the mind, but the physical mechanism thereof, the body's functional organ that facilitates the workings of the mind.

And researching the workings of the neural pathways and its chemical messengers (neuropeptides) follows in the wake of this. Early on, a doctor directed me to the book Molecules of Emotion – Candace Pert (Pocketbooks; 1997). This scientist proved the connection between emotions and the working of chemical messengers in the brain, which explains more than the obvious (depression).

The SPECT research of Dr. Daniel Amen cast even more light on how the brain functions are affected by chemical changes (Change your brain, change your life)(1999).

Candace Pert did her research in the early 1970s to prove the biochemical nature of brain function. She embarked upon studies that led to the discovery of neuropeptides, fuelled initially by the search for the opiate receptor in the brain. Her research has led to the discovery that neuropeptides are also present in the intestinal tract, the endocrine system and the immune systems, in fact they are present throughout the body. She refers to these peptides as the "molecules of emotion".

Pert found that viruses use the same receptors to get into a cell that peptides do. This explains why people with a happier disposition do not get sick as often as their more melancholic friends. The receptors are kept occupied by feel-good substances like endorphins and thus viruses cannot find entry into the cells. It also explains why two people confronted with the same viral load may react differently – one perhaps becoming very ill and the other not ill at all. This also explains why I feel energized and refreshed after a run!

Pert regarded the emotions as cellular signals involved in translating information into physical reality. "Emotions are the nexus between matter and mind, going back and forth between the two and influencing both," she wrote.

It follows then that illness also influences emotions, just like the reverse. And chronic pain, which demands the suppression of emotions and giving vent to feelings, most certainly will lead to negative emotions, setting up a vicious circle of illness affecting emotions and emotions affecting illness.

According to Dr. Pert: "Emotions are what unite the mind and body. Anger, fear and sadness (negative emotions) are as healthy as peace, courage and joy. To repress these emotions and not let them flow freely is to set up a dis-integrity in the system, causing it to act at cross-purposes rather than as a unified whole. The stress this causes which takes the form of blockages and insufficient flow of peptide signals to maintain functions at the cellular level is what sets up the weakened condition that can lead to disease. " The long-held belief in energy blockages in the Chakras come to mind...

Minefield in the Mind

The minefield in the mind has kept me busy ever since that fateful day that I woke up dead. That small pinpoint of darkness which has come to stay in my soul (or has it always been there, and I only recognized it at this time in my life?) has been the source of daily questioning – year in and year out.

John Milton said "The mind is its own place, and in itself can make a heaven of hell, and a hell of heaven."

If you think this book is about how my overriding will to live led me back to health, it is not. It is much more about the struggle against this small but significant blackness that had me asking to die, not striving to live, for more years than I can remember.

Thanatos, post-Freudians called it, based on his idea of the force opposing the life force. The fact that within you there is both the will to live and the will to die. Some may think I am referring to being suicidal. I am not suicidal and have never been.

As a person who firmly believes there is a better life after this one, with God, I do hold to the idea that it would be better to die, but of course, I will never find peace in the idea of taking my own life. That however, does not touch what I am referring to here. How strong are the forces in one's own soul, the one to live and the other to die? This unwelcome dichotomy still has to find a peaceable place in my soul.

And then you have to work at finding enough meaning to stay alive while wanting not to be. Personally, I have not found meaning other than the life of my fatherless child. That, one might say, is enough.

The purpose-led life

The very much-publicized idea that each person should be living the plan for his (her) life? After years of soul searching I have reached the point where I believe that some of us will never know what the meaning of their life is supposed to be. A purpose-driven life… really. We are all reading the stuff and believing we should have what it tells us we should have, should live in the way it propounds. I do not doubt that for some, who slavishly gulps up everything they read, it works. But perhaps getting through a day with love and the satisfaction of not having done another person harm, is meaning enough.

If you can map out your life in years, in chunks or whatever, you could possibly define such a purpose that drives you. But I lost that ability when I lay sick in bed with nothing to cling to, not even the will to live. Next week, even tomorrow, became a vague concept, not a possible reality. I could not plan. Not even a week ahead. Since I have regained my health, this goal-setting, driven lifestyle has still not become a reality for me.

I do plan things, of course I do. But not years or months in advance. Every day of my life is planned with military precision, but that holds to my calling around, reading up, and setting the bar in what I see as a rare sight: a truly caring doctor.

One friend recounted her experience with her family GP who insisted she was suffering from depression… and the more she refuted this one-dimensional, over-simplistic diagnosis, the less he listened and insisted on giving her a script for an antidepressant.

He followed this up with a phone call to her parents, telling them that she was refusing to listen to him. She was far from being a child, if I recall she was already in her thirties… how unprofessional. She did follow my suggestion that she report him to the medical professional council, who took it up with him immediately. Perhaps this gave her some satisfaction, but unfortunately it did nothing to improve her health!

I have had some doctors telling me ME was just a dinner party topic and not a disease condition. This they did while the WHO had already classified it as a disease of the central nervous system. My anger stems from this lack of interest, this lack of knowledge from professionals who should know about the disease. At the same time as hearing this comment, medical aids in South Africa refused to extend cover to patients over whom the cloud called ME was hovering… a paradox the unemployed, ill, patient found very, very difficult to deal with.

Blaming the patient

The medical fraternity *in toto* has created this situation where they blame the patient for being ill, by treating them in this way. The mere fact that ME is not a fatal disease does not mean patients are less ill than others with infectious or fatal diseases. And proof says that ME can be triggered by an infection or even multiple infections. Too many times have I seen the attitude among doctors and nurses that they actually know everything and since they don't know what to say to you, you are not really ill, and to blame for whatever is wrong with you. Never have I seen ME patients given the care and empathy that cancer patients receive – in fact, a large dose of disrespect is more often the norm.

Anger and disgust became quite common emotions to me, as I tried to stay positive amidst the worst experience of my life... with physical pain blotting out my thought processes. Earlier in my life I had quite a number of experiences with pain... quite a few operations for bunions, gallbladder, appendix, and the like. But in all these instances the pain eventually left. And I became pain-free even though I had experienced something bad.

Now, pain had become my constant companion, and one I wished to rid myself of. Some years down the line, as editor of a medical publication, I visited a rheumatologist and was discussing rheumatological diseases with him. He told me of a man in his eighties with rheumatoid arthritis who expressed the thought that he would rather die than live every day with the debilitating, progressive disease which had him in such pain that his quality of life was very, very low. Oh boy... I could relate to that so well because I had fought that battle with constant pain for years on end, with no-one giving me support, no medical answers, no pill or potion to relieve my thoughts from being centered entirely on the pain in my body.

Regaining control

Looking back I can accept that negative emotions played more than one role in the disease process: on the one hand it holds you back from getting better and on the other hand it was a causative factor in itself. Yes, emotions can make you ill. It can make you better too.

Pain, unfortunately has the power to override your thoughts to the point where emotions become secondary to the experience of pain. It does not matter where in the body the pain is, if its intensity is this high, it becomes your master. And regaining control of your thoughts and your emotions is far from easy.

How to do it? Is there one easy answer? Perhaps the answer is that one needs to become conscious of this fact. The very realization that you need to take back control is the starting point. As Dr. Phil has taught the world, you cannot change what you do not acknowledge. Thus realizing that pain is in control of you and that you need to take control of your own self, your own body, and of course, your own thoughts is the starting point.

What a mammoth task. There are many books on this subject... quite a few borderline ones too. Some are 'woo-woo' (my own description of things that are outside the boundaries and falling off the esoteric radar) and others are thinly-veiled attempts to sell books. Mind control, or mind power, as a topic, has been made popular by people like John Kehoe. That the mind controls your being, including your body, has been known since Bible days.

Might I pop a thought in here? Every person will arrive at this point from his own reference framework. Some may reject certain things out of hand based on their religious beliefs. My journey of discovery started here. Based on what I believed, I was a wary traveler, even before I became a weary traveler.

There are many truths out there. And what you do about it, which truth you embrace, is your own choice. Take care though, some things will lead you down the wrong path. But let's get back to the basic truth that your mind controls your life. And that your thoughts determine what happens on all levels. Most of us grow up without ever realizing that we can take control of the millions of thoughts running through our minds – and that we should accept responsibility for it.

Another battlefield

This is a constant battle. Research has tried to pin down the number of thoughts running through the average person's mind during the course of a day – and can only indicate that it numbers in the thousands upon thousands, perhaps in the hundreds of thousands. Sure, we do know that you do not think only one thought at a time, followed by another .. but taking control of the many simultaneous thoughts?

This is not easy. Yet, remember that, even if you don't feel like it, you can change the course of your thoughts. You can make a difference. You may not sense control but you can change this, one step at a time. Remember thoughts are not experienced in a linear continuum but as lots of disjointed thoughts, which join together when they find similarities – like a bowl of spaghetti.

My experience runs to unbidden visual pictures popping into my mind, such as a picture of me sitting on a bus in Rome. These are mostly memories, but not all. What does it mean? I have no idea. Perhaps I am longing to be somewhere else. Or maybe it means something I have yet to discover. I often will see these pictures in my mind, of things that seem random and not linked to anything I am thinking.

But I do react to thoughts that pop into my mind unbidden, especially if they are negative. Sad thoughts in particular, are with me most of my waking moments. Loss has been with me since I lost my father when I was twenty. The shock of his sudden death took me years to work through. And after the shock I have been left with the loss. More than thirty years later, I think of him every day. Miss him every day, and feel sad about this loss every day. Many other losses have added to this over the years. And every new loss breaks loose the devastation I experienced when I lost him.

But I have had to learn not to let the sadness control my thoughts, or my life. Pushing the thoughts away is not enough, though. Being in control means, from my experience, to be able to embrace the thoughts, allow them room to breathe, and to let them go. I remember being told as a child not to think 'like that', or not to feel a certain emotion. This does not work. One person cannot tell another how to think or feel. What this insistence of a parent does to a child is to teach him/her to suppress feelings and thoughts. This is both negative and destructive. It teaches the child that he should not express emotion.

Pretending is fake

Always pretending and not being true to one's emotions can lead to major problems if this continues year after year. The term passive-aggressive pops into my mind. If you are not allowed to show how you feel, and suppress your feelings until you are alone, it means that you fail to address the sources of your discontent and walk away pretending that everything is fine, while they are not. It also teaches one to shy away from confrontation, which is negative in itself. It teaches you that you should remain quiet and submissive in all situations.

Apart from not teaching you to cope with reality, it creates internal problems which, on their own, down the line need long years of hard work to correct.

Therefore, imagine being treated badly by a nurse. You feel angry, but you dare not express it. (If you do, they brush you aside and refuse to help you. Really, they do. They are really aware of the power they wield). Month after month, visit after visit, the anger builds and becomes a destructive emotional drain on your fatigued self.

I have read the advice numerous times over the years, to rid yourself of toxic people, or toxic relationships. This is easier said than done! You cannot simply avoid all negative things – you would not leave your house or even switch on the television, in fact even in monasteries (where peace should reign) negative people or situations are unavoidable.

More relevant is the ability to not allow negativity to drag you down. As I have said already, it is not just a case of pushing it away, it is a case of, even when you are affected by it, being able to put a boundary down and refuse to allow the negativity to cross the boundary. Life is not all wine and roses. If it was, we would all be drunkards! It cannot ever be positive all the time. You have to be able to stop the loose strands of negativity from becoming a negative force. If you are in a conversation that is dragging you down and cannot leave, make up your mind to not allow the negativity to attach itself to you.

Some people preach positivity as if it is a cure-all drug. They deny the negative – but without negative force the universe would cease to exist. Then there is the "balance" belief – that everything should be in balance – like the yin and yang belief. I do not hold to this. To me it is more like a continuous give and take between the two. Life is an ebb and flow of thoughts, feelings and events, both negative and positive.

Denying – or repressing – an emotion does not make it disappear, instead, it causes a steady build-up that will, at some point, demand being defused. This is usually a crisis point, one which the people around the detonating dummy can hardly believe, not to mention understand. Many couples end in big fights with the one partner not understanding how they got to this point. It took me some years to figure this out about myself...

At the same time, allow yourself times of negativity, sadness or feeling more down than up, and learn to put the brakes on in time. In other words, feeling blue is okay as long as you don't wallow. Wallowing can become a habit – and the habit can become addictive.

A few thoughts on research into ME (or any illness for that matter) while being ill. As described already, medical staff are not the ones with answers... and all the ME sufferers I have met, have had to embark on their own quest to discover answers and find relief. I fell ill before the internet became part of our lives and therefore had to find information in the library. I did find information as there were a few books on the topic already.

Now, however, the internet with its fingertip-ready information allows for both the positive and negative in this regard. Reading and researching to find answers and treatment options, can lead a person into psychological dungeons. It may make you feel more helpless, more hopeless, less in control, as it can also do the opposite. Depending on the person and his state of mind, it may make him sicker than before because it could be overwhelming. It is a fine line to negotiate.

Dr. Collinge in his book Recovering from ME, (GP Putnam and Sons, 1993) uses the analogy of carrying a heavy suitcase, which requires the body to compensate on the opposite side of the weight. This is a good depiction of how a person has to adapt to having symptoms and pain. But it also, as he

The problem is, these verses are quoted out of context. Imagine, the salutation of a letter, being used as a hanging peg for a doctrine: 3 John 2 "Beloved, I wish that you should prosper and be in good health." Like making a law out of saying "Hi.. hope you are well".

I have in the following years become quite averse to Bible verses being quoted willy nilly and out of context, for obvious reasons. However, it is also a matter of **spiritual growth**. I myself would quote at any moment, without thinking, Bible verses that sounded like answers to things people would be talking about.

In the same way, little verses being pulled from a tiny container, could well encourage people in a general sense, but taken out of context may well be either meaningless or could be construed to mean just about anything a person would like to read into it.. this practice is not so far removed from a card reader peering into a deck of cards and saying something general like: "things will get better for you within the next couple of weeks", leaving you to fill in the blanks, so to speak.

Encouragement

Don't imagine that there were no people I found encouragement from — there were those who acknowledged their lack of understanding and yet encouraged me. But the larger group of Christians were harshly condemning my illness and failing to extend to me anything resembling the love of Christ.

Self-denial. I grew up in a timeframe and a home that forcibly sustained this belief that everyone else's needs should be put before one's own. A really nice Christian principle. Question is, how does self-denial play into a negative self-image, lack of self-esteem and the like? If you have low self-esteem it follows that you have low self-respect too. And this self-image that you project into the world, becomes a self-fulfilling prophecy as others treat you like a lowly serf since you denigrate yourself and perpetuate being treated badly by others.

Then the eighties hit us with this concept of self-realization – where each had to reach the heights of self-fulfillment and achieve all there is to grab on the way to the top, where the focus was not on denying, but on promoting yourself.

I have seen that people, instead of respecting and thanking you for thinking ahead and smoothing their path in the act of self-denial, trample over you on their way to the top without as much as a backward (or downward, as may be) glance. And if you are stupid enough to think anyone would thank you for your efforts – you are to be disappointed all along the way. More than any other thing in my life, being brought up in this way, naïvely believing people to be generally good, this has shocked me – especially in so-called Christians. I have seen more self-serving Christians than what I would like to have known.

Churches like to preach self-denial. And yet I have seen in more than one church set-up people walking over others to whom they preach this principle – as if using it as a weapon while getting their own way in the name of Jesus.

How does self-denial turn into disease? Pert quotes Linda Temoshok who showed that cancer patients who repressed their emotions had slower rates of recovery. Self-denial stems from unawareness of one's own emotional needs and suppressing these needs chips away at the immune system, as shown by work done with cancer patients in the 1980s. Freud, more than a century ago, already called depression anger directed at oneself. This view is being proved to be scientifically and chemically true.

Pert says that the stress of repressing emotions creates blockages and insufficient flow of peptide signals to maintain the correct flow at the cellular level, which sets up the weakened conditions leading to disease.

Chapter Eleven

Victim or survivor?

Becoming ill makes one a victim. This is unavoidable. Whether you remain a victim and succumb to all the negatives the illness imposes on you, will be determined by a series of choices. And the point where you change from being a victim to being a survivor may well not be a recognizable event, or turning point in the play on the stage of your life – it might just be a place on the continuum of life as you live it.

How many people actually live their lives being totally connected and tuned in at every stage during every day? We spend most of our day repeating rituals without consciously regarding what we are doing. We get up, switch the light on, boil the kettle for tea, and so on, till we put our heads on our pillows at night and switch the light off, without our minds being part of the majority of the processes we go through in our day.

Thus what goes on in our lives on the subconscious level, orchestrates the nitty-gritty grind of activities we have to undertake. And also in the subconscious lies our belief systems, the blueprints according to which we think ourselves through our lives.

How you think about being ill, about your life being disrupted and changed to a grinding Ferris wheel of painful difficulty, depends on your personal reference framework. People from eastern countries have vastly different beliefs when it comes to disease.

I am sorry to say that the Western way of thinking when it comes to sickness and health has already proven to fail most people who present with problems other than single-pathogen infections and disease conditions that have decades (or centuries) of studies behind them.

But even in an overall sense, we have been brought up to think that you go through life until you fall ill – when you go to a doctor, who will sort the problem out, in the first instance with a script, or if more serious, with surgical intervention.

External attack?

This has led us to not even think about our health until we are forced to think about it. Fortunately, over the past two decades this has changed a lot – although mostly just in the sense of people being more aware of their own health and taking more responsibility by trying to live healthier lives (this is only true of a portion of the population anyway).

Eastern belief sees the body and mind as a connected whole and the body-mind concept has filtered into many alternative (complementary) health systems, such as Body Talk which embraces many different systems into an integrated (holistic) system.

But let's consider first how you think of contracting an infection. Do you see the pathogen as being from outside and having invaded your body? What about inflammation? Does this come from outside, or inside? Allergies? This is an immune response so therefore comes from inside, does it not? The allergen may be from outside but the response is from inside…

Some may postulate that illness is an attack (spiritual/mental) which has to be warded off outside the body. Some others believe that it is demonic/satanic and that the person should be "delivered". (Actually, I did go for "deliverance" but no demon manifested…)

On the other hand, other belief systems hold that the body is in dis-ease, and therefore the body's own systems should be attended to for healing to take place. Think of the system of chakras in the Buddhist and Hindu belief systems which says that obstruction of the energy flow in the body will cause disease.

If you think you can ward off the illness with mind power, once again your belief is based on the assumption that illness is something outside which you have to fight from inside your mind.

On a cellular level, you may think of the damage a virus has caused inside the cell, resulting in the cell changing its normal functioning. Thus we have something from outside, causing problems once it is inside your body. This probably holds true for most Western minds' thinking.

But why is thinking about the disease important? Why not just pop the pills and get on with your life? Many years ago my GP would give me a script for an antibiotic to fight off an infection, and instruct me to stay home. This I blithely disregarded every time, citing the reason as not being able to stay off work… because no-one else would take care of my workload.

Turning the tide

When becoming severely ill, the doctor who helped me turn the tide on ME, stressed that rest is 70% of recovery… and I always refused to take even a day off. Now I can kick myself. What does it matter if something gets done a day later? In the greater scheme of things, this day of rest, had I taken it when I should have, might have changed the course of my life years down the line…!

But I did not listen. I just lived my life at close to break-neck speed with little thought as to the possible consequences. And pay the price I did. In many more ways than just losing my health. I also lost my career, and many relationships suffered irreparably. Too bad, one might say. And truthfully, I do not think of it and mourn the loss of people who did not see their way open to remain in my circle. What would be the point? But I have not forgotten how their responses and reactions – and consequent actions, have hurt me, much more than I ever admitted at the time.

This is also why I am single and will most likely remain so. After more than 30 years of being alone I have come to accept that it is most likely the only way to remain sane. And not having to apologize for what I have become. I live my life on a level that other people do not always understand. And in many instances I really do not care what they think.

Yet sometimes I long for some understanding from others, but when I have tried to explain to some people, I have met with dead stares and incomprehension which left me wondering why I had even bothered. I have come to believe only a person who has had to deal with chronic pain or a disease condition can relate to another going through similar adversity.

One of the many things I have learned is that you have to expend some of your "brain energy" just to get through a day. In other words, you have to actively think in the moment, of what you are doing, those actions usually performed by the body in an unconscious way, you have to consciously put into place.

Similarly, chronic pain drains your energy by necessitating your mind to push the pain down into the subconscious.

Dealing with chronic pain

When your body refuses to heal, when the pain refuses to lift, feeling depressed is inevitable. This is reactive depression, not clinical depression. And, as I said, inevitable. Who can remain upbeat and happy, singing with joy, while experiencing debilitating pain?

And from some quarters the unrelenting pressure: be joyful, be happy, be healed... this does nothing to make you even the slightest bit better.

The pain that had me in its grip for the greater part of fifteen years, was initially generalized in all my large skeletal muscles. Drying my hair was agony. Walking was difficult and standing the worst activity of all. It took me a long time to figure out that my standing problem was due to orthostatic hypotension.

Of course, standing in a queue was the most dreadful thing I had to do. No-one could explain that within a short space of time I would become really dizzy and had to hold onto something just to remain upright. Needless to say no-one around me at such times would believe that I was really dizzy; they would rather think that I was trying to jump the queue!

In the beginning I tried to find answers to the pain. That was after the fatigue lifted enough for my brain to start functioning. My leg muscles were stiff and sore. At the same time as burning, it also felt numb.

When they saw me I held on to every shred of my almost defunct dignity and hoped to look normal even though I did not feel it. The duality of this is something I want to highlight here.

Think of the internal stress this creates. Pretense. Having to pretend to feel fine, drains your brain energy. I gave up trying to participate and eventually did nothing but sit quietly and nodding at certain intervals. Yet at the end of such interaction I suffered the consequences by being utterly floored with fatigue and having to find recovery time just to get my body up and working again.

Reaching beyond the pain and staying involved in life is a challenge in its own right.

Chapter Twelve

Does the way your doctor treats you have an effect on your recovery?

The answer to this question is a resounding yes. And when all is said and done, one wonders how medical schools qualify doctors with little or no understanding of the psychology of being a medical practitioner. In years long gone there was a noticeable "white coat" phenomenon: patients whose blood pressure rose in response to the white coat, in other words, they had a psychological response to the setting.. and the doctor's white coat exacerbated it to the extent where physiological responses could be measured.

Eastern philosophies and religions, and their medical practices, have examined things that we are now beginning to prove beyond reasonable doubt to be true about the mind and body and their connection and interaction.

Westerners, on the other hand, have been brought up in a paradigm where we believe doctors to be all-powerful and have all the answers.

I have read many times about Norman Cousins and "how he laughed himself out of an illness". If you read his own version of what happened to him, you see clearly that much more was at work in his situation. He stated unequivocally that having had a doctor who was open-minded and listened to him, and supported his suggestions about treatment, even though it would have seemed outrageous at that time, was what allowed his return to health from a debilitating condition which, according to specialists, would have seen him dead.

Cousins did his own research and made suggestions to his doctor which was put into practice. Thus the laughter was one of a few contributors. The other was intravenous ascorbic acid (vitamin C). By the way I had a few Vitamin C drips also – and can personally attest to the good response my body had to this.

But let us consider the need for a diagnosis. A very ill patient who had given up on helping himself, will go to the doctor looking for answers and help to get better. Depending on the doctor his recovery may be swift, or delayed. (I have wondered whether doctors consciously treat patients in a way that will ensure their return – in other words, making sure they don't recover immediately.) Sounds perverse, but perhaps there is even more than just a grain of truth in it.

I have mentioned some instances elsewhere of how I have been treated by doctors. Let us in summary look at some examples.

The hostile hammer

This doctor is not always identifiable at a glance. Sometimes it takes some time before he shows his true colors. He may even be softly spoken at first. But at some point during the appointment, he becomes hostile and hammers you with questions and incredulous looks, scoffing at your words, and being downright negative.

No patient has ever been helped in this way... not that I know of. Patients who feel helpless will upon been mistreated in this way, turn from doctors altogether. This might not be such a bad thing!

I am aware that patients too, come in different shapes and sizes, and emotional make-up. When will doctors start to evaluate their patients in terms of what they are like as people? After all the patient is a human being with a body AND a mind. And a psyche that is taking a beating when confronted by a difficult-to-treat illness.

If the complaint is less than debilitating or less serious, such as an everyday infection sure to clear up, even when accompanied by symptoms such as a severe cough, the patient's state of mind would be more positive and therefore, a less than helpful, unfriendly doctor would do little damage in this scenario. But a patient whose energy is depleted, who feels helpless and drained, will be left with a feeling of disgust. The little flicker of hope that was present before walking into the doctor's consulting room would be doused and the feeling of hopelessness would again be growing, instead of diminishing.

Helpful Hannah

This GP is one who sees the patient as more than just a bag of symptoms, and even if stumped by what she is confronted with, remains helpful and intent on changing the patient's scenario. Many Helpful Hannahs welcome input from their patients, and consider factors other than pure physiological ones, as part of the disease process.

Some Hannahs eventually throw in the towel, with a shrug and a shake of the head. They often offer to write a script for whatever you suggest. This, from the perspective of a person who has studied and continues to study the disease and the body and its psychological components, is not really a bad thing. However, this could well be a cop-out that could at best be OK and perhaps even cause damage to some patients.

Scriptwriter Sam

The archetypal traditional doctor in a brand new guise... who grabs the prescription pad after a mere two minutes of discussion and pen in hand, will put up a show of listening to you, even though seasoned patients will know that the doctor is aching to write the script and get rid of him at the earliest opportunity.

Scriptwriter Sam is conditioned to think in terms of drugs. His being is ensconced in treatment paradigms, and he sees little beyond the presentation of a set of symptoms, which he tries to synthesize into a picture fitting his known treatment paradigms and send the patient off with a sympathetic pat on the back.

Scoffing Samantha

Unfortunately by the time you realize that you are with one of these, they have already taken your payment (upfront). One of the many examples I can cite, is that of a neurologist who, at my first (and only) visit, failed to even do a proper examination, and while taking notes on my history, I tried to give a full account of the situation.

I mentioned to her that my GP who referred me to her, had on occasion used a certain injection (cortisone) and that I had experienced some relief from it. She paused and looked at me and her response was: "If you want injections, go somewhere else, I don't give injections". I wanted, and still want, my money back from this insult to the medical profession. Doctors like this should not practice medicine. All she did was scoff at what I was saying and I had to pay her for this privilege. And there are many of them out there.

Cousins writes in his book about a woman who wrote to him that she asked her doctor about the ascorbic acid treatment, and her doctor actually making sounds going "quack quack". A scoffing Sam, who deserved to lose his patient, perhaps many of his patients.

Persistent Pete

My favorite, and as scarce as hen's teeth. This kind of GP will not let go, will persevere and try every avenue to help a patient... beyond the norm. I have met three such doctors in my time. You know the doctor is earnest when he calls you up after the visit, having read up on things you mentioned and taking the time to investigate the things he had not encountered before.

ME when it had its first round in the full glare of the media, confused doctors and patients alike. Today the literature is there, the scientific proof of many differential diagnoses has been published, but without a GP who persists to the point where he helps the individual patient with his particular set of symptoms (and underlying causes) the patient still founders on a bed of pain without much hope.

One factor that sets Petes apart from their colleagues is the willingness to listen. Helpful Hannahs are also good with this. But the Petes persist and this goes into looking at ALL factors of the patient's circumstances, including life situations, stress factors, financial factors, et all. And the other important distinguishing factor is Petes' ability to accept input from the patient on things he has tried, literature he has read, and suggestions as to what can be tried next. For way too long doctors have shunned the very true statement that no one knows a person's body better than himself.

I have a huge measure of respect for Persistent Pete doctors. They know how to approach a person holistically, and when they hit a wall in their search for answers, they would confess it, yet are not deterred. One doctor I know, aware of my financial situation, went out of his way to contact others and enlist their help. In my memory he is the only one that had gone to such lengths to help me.

Desperation feeds depression

Very few doctors have shown an understanding of the fact that being desperately ill will make you feel depressed, eventually. That the very brushes with the medical fraternity presented a negative element which, if you feel powerless to start with, will add to your feelings of being powerless, and make you feel depressed because you lose hope.

This does not mean that you suffer from clinical depression... but that you are experiencing reactive depression, as a result of your life situation.

These are distinct entities, and for those who want to grab the antidepressants, well, I have right from the start shunned the idea of a chemical that will do little other than mask what is there and should be attended to.

What would be the point to start taking a drug which might be habit-forming, which does not begin to address the underlying cause of the disease, has always been my stance on this. As for depression, I sometimes feel depressed, but I see life as a series of highs and lows. Those who believe one should always be on a high, positive and coruscating, are damaging the essence of the life we have been given. This is simply not natural. It is not summer year-round… winter comes along in season.

Feeling depressed will follow hopelessness and helplessness. Following from my earlier thoughts on doctors, how much could be done if doctors were to focus on giving patients hope. How uplifting that would be. As I have mentioned, from the Hostile Hammer to Scriptwriter Sam, a very large percentage of doctors see their patients as a presentation of a set of symptoms that they approach scientifically.

Remember the scene in Patch Adams where the ambulating group trudges on their rounds around the ward and stops at a patient who is referred to only by her medical condition? In fact, the very message of this movie rests on the change in symptoms and even disease progression, when patients are treated like humans instead of scientific sets of data.

I have often thought about that which the movie sets out to depict, and what Patch articulates as "treating the patient, not the disease". Why do doctors - those of a persistent nature, and those who start with good intentions - not take their eyes off writing a script and rather concentrate on improving a patient's quality of life?

In his impassioned speech in front of hundreds of his peers Patch said the worst disease of all is indifference. He stumbled on the truth that the brought to bear the idea that nothing was as potent as the state of mind that a patient brings to his disease.

Suffice to say: doctors can do severe damage!

Chapter 13

The process of illness

Why do you need to understand the process of illness? You need to synthesize this understanding into your holistic life experience to be able to make sense of what you are, who you have become, what you have to try and regain and how you have to redefine yourself. Illness creates suffering and suffering, as Frankl pointed out " completely fills the human soul and conscious mind, no matter whether great or little, the size of human suffering is absolutely relative."

Letting go of what you have lost. Initially I tried to hang on: to friendships, to beliefs, to my life as it used to be. This was a futile exercise. Of course being unable to sit upright for more than half an hour was proving untenable. Even attending church was simply not possible (our services tended to run over two hours at a time).

Friendships suffered a lot and some went out the door. Those who remained, are the ones I cherish to this day. Being a friend to someone even if you do not quite understand what is happening, is difficult. From my perspective, I did not expect others to understand – since I did not understand most of it myself! In time, though, I gained understanding and could articulate it quite well – but eventually stopped trying to, simply because I felt it was a boring topic. Yes, indeed, sick people do not want to talk about their illness all the time and some become quite embarrassed when questioned relentlessly about body functions, pain and its future outlook.

Freedom from wrong beliefs

And as for hanging onto my beliefs, this is what the illness did for me: it set me free from faulty beliefs, in a major way. Being analytical by nature, I am inclined to do mountains of research before ascribing to something.

On the spiritual level, of course, this is not how it goes. One becomes convinced of something without having done the research. And if you are in a situation where everything and everyone around you perpetuate the belief/s, and in a severe "knuckle under" type of scenario... in which the overall understanding was clear: if the pastor says it is so, it is. And you have to accept without question his leadership over you.

Might I add that apart from the spiritual implications of this on a personal level I suffered incredible damage due to this, on which I would rather not elucidate?

I managed, even though it took years to accomplish, to re-evaluate, re-investigate and re-define myself, my beliefs and, I hope, my spiritual and mental well-being.

The first I let go was my expectations of life in general. This is obvious due to physical limitations that enforces this even against your will. But more significantly, the beliefs I had built my life on – based on the Bible, came under intense scrutiny and as I investigated and researched the basis of these doctrines, I let go of most of them.

Without explaining in detail, I have come to understand the problems arising from building your life on faulty beliefs. I still love the Lord and will never stop doing so, but approach the interpretation of His Word cautiously these days.

Looking back on life, I faced the fact that I had lived through a series of possibilities which turned into a long line of realities, which include the joys of days past and the sufferings that have come my way. I love what Dostoevsky said about it: "there is only one thing I dread: not being worthy of my suffering". Yet, as Frankl pointed out no–one envies you your sufferings; why would they? He also wistfully mentioned viewing suffering as achievement and accomplishment. In our post-modern society we reach out to some who achieve something against all odds. Yet this happens only on a superficial plane and does not reach right down into the depths where thousands are caught in their personal sufferings.

The courage to suffer

Who was it that framed the question: "do you have the courage to suffer?" This I find quite a good question. The answer though is one you will only discover when the suffering slips its cape over you and refuses to let go. Before you know it the cape turns into an octopus that wraps its tentacles around you sucking onto your body with determination and persistence. However, as Nietzsche so poignantly pointed out, what does not kill you, makes you stronger.

Have you ever considered the inner strength gained from chronic disease? When looking at a person lying in a bed, hooked up to machines, do you ask yourself what immense inner strength suffering demands? That person has to reach into his innermost being to find courage for every moment he remains alive in that bed. He has to find joy somewhere – which others can derive from being able to live their lives in the way they choose to: to participate in sport, climb mountains or go dancing. Pleasure, enjoyment, joy... this does not come at a price when you can reach out and take it.

Joy, on the other hand, is a hard-won commodity for a chronic pain sufferer. It is a lesson that takes a long time to learn; how to find joy amid pain and suffering. Some people do not manage to find it, as can be seen in old age homes and hospitals where some patients are cranky, miserable and even downright disagreeable. They have lost their joy altogether and finding it may even be beyond their reach.

No-one can take your experiences away from you, or replace them with others!

The losing game

Before falling ill, I had already suffered the most significant loss in my life: my father. I have now lived more years than what I had spent with him in my life. Only time taught me the real value of the loss. He was gone before I could build a relationship with him. And that loss had a lot to do with subsequent choices I made: most of them questionable, or downright bad.

Falling ill though, brought a slew of losses in its wake. This is one factor doctors fail to address, I think. In my case, very few of them considered the fact that I had no income. When stumped by the fact that I could not pay for expensive medical tests and in some cases, exotic treatment, they just gave up with a shrug of their shoulders. I have, thankfully, experienced the opposite as well.

Loss of a job, loss of income. And the loss of a career which was on an upward path. Loss of energy, loss of joy, loss of light. Ultimately, battling a waning self-image, and the final fight to not lose my faith in myself.

But faith in myself, in my abilities – those abilities I no longer had – that was the ultimate test. Even now this is an up and down daily battle waging in my mind and soul. I know what I am capable of – intellectually and analytically. Yet, due to my long absence from the job market, I am now eating the crumbs of others' tables, having to make do with entry-level jobs and concomitant low incomes, while I am fully capable as a middle-weight manager. How to make the jump from the bottom to the middle? In a job market that favors others who have not had my disadvantages? I don't have the answer.

Loss on another level: the loss of love. Somewhere during the early recovery phase I met a man – a beautiful one. For him, I felt love such as none other I had ever felt before or since. I truly believed that God had put him in my life. That together we were going to fulfill God's purpose. Until one day we were having coffee in a shopping center in Johannesburg… and sensing something was off-kilter, I asked him if something was wrong.

He had been putting his children between us for weeks – not talking to me directly and I picked up on him distancing himself. Well, the moment of truth came and hit me in my face when he told me point blank that he could not deal with my illness and wanted to end our relationship. That shook my faith in God – I won't even discuss, against this backdrop, what it did to my faith in myself.

Unfortunately one reaches a place where you are defined by the disease. It not only defines your lifestyle, your income (or lack thereof), it defines who you are, how you think and how you see yourself. My self-image (albeit realistic) was very far from complimentary. I have always been a true realist, seeing things in a stark, non-blurred way. Fuzzy edges meant fuzzy logic to me – which did not work for hyper-analytical individuals such as myself.

Then there were the days when you nurtured the stupid idea that you were healed – healthy – thinking yourself invincible – beyond the pain and illness. Then the next infection took hold and you were once again horizontally contemplating the sunset, which would indicate that you had lived another day.

You found once again that you are not invincible or even protected against the pathogens which seek to besiege your cells. And thus: back to basics. How to get up, and stay up, when your body drags you down. And coping with the thought that you were wrong: you were not healed, and still in the battle against pain and disease.

In the fifty-plus years of my life I have had a preponderance of days when my body did not feel up to getting through the long stretch of hours in a day, and where my brain had to be forced by my mind and my (often reluctant) determination to get through the day. How many days have I had to force myself to face the day while my body screamed at me that it was not able to do so? I have no idea, but I imagine it is close to being in the majority since I was forced to start this battle with illness.

Coming to terms with loss is inextricably linked with re-defining yourself. You have to accept what you have lost, and that you have lost it (them) and move along to a new place where you replace the loss with something else. There is no time frame for this. Some things are easier to accept and deal with than others. And, as AA teaches in its 12-step program, it is a matter of taking things one day at a time.

Chapter Fourteen

The road to rediscovery

To rediscover implies that you have made your discoveries already, such as those I had made for myself on the way to my 34th birthday. I thought I had life sussed, really I did. I had things pretty clear (in my mind) and quite sure of what I thought relating to the things I dealt with, and thought of, during the course of a day in my life.

At the time of falling down fatigued to the point of not getting up again, in my 34th year on this earth, I was a raving charismatic Christian. I was in fact, on a stint as a missionary when this happened to me. Try putting yourself in that spot: where the church to whose beliefs you subscribe, believe that Christians cannot be sick, and you unable to walk, or function.

Several months later I was on an outreach where I played the keyboard non-stop for six hours without sitting down once. When I then asked to return home to rest, a fellow Christian came up to me and said point-blank that he has a problem with me having a disease.

"Christians cannot be sick," he said. "Your sickness is embarrassing to us".

He suggested that I get a set of tapes on healing by Kenneth Copeland or Hagin, I can't remember which. He said that his family listen to these tapes every day and that not one of them has been sick since. Well, that's all good and well. I brushed him off but was thinking to myself: do I now have to take lower-rung jobs because you have lost years of your life, the longing to be able to do what you used to, becomes acute.

My creativity has been stifled for years and years. While in my mind I know that I have talents and creative drive, I have not, due to falling ill, advanced my career and am now stuck in a place where I suffer frustration on a minute-to-minute basis.

Frankl talks about being brave, dignified and unselfish in the midst of suffering. I try to be all of those, but the frustration sometimes weigh so heavy I literally feel my knees buckling under the strain. And thus, another question: why was I made with creative and other talents, if I cannot actually use them?

Years down the line, looking back I realize that I had developed my own unique form of *intangible creativity* in the plans I had to come up with to stay alive, to create my own work and income, and in fact, to get through a day. This was not creativity that wowed other people... but it attributed to me staying alive daily and managing to live through every day that I have been given.

I sometimes wonder whether all people experience this constant quest for answers that drives my every waking moment. In talking to someone recently, he pointed to the fact that not everything has a logical explanation (especially seen from a spiritual perspective). Yes, I am still battling with questions that plagued me twenty years ago. But I am not the person I was then. I have died to that person, and have very few memories to hang my hat on. Thus what I was contemplating twenty years ago had undergone a major shift in understanding and interpretation.

Frankl says the meaning of life lies in saying **yes to life *despite*** everything. Life is potentially meaningful under any conditions, even the most miserable. This he clearly saw in Auschwitz. He concluded that once an individual's search for meaning is successful, it not only renders him happy but also gives him the capability to cope with suffering.

He also pointed to one of the most profound truths of all time: "everything can be taken from a man but one thing: to choose his attitude in a given set of circumstances". Some have pointed to this as the definition of freedom. Did Nelson Mandela not illustrate this to the benefit of an entire country? Choosing one attitude above another, he changed the course of history.

Is this not where most people fall off the bus? Media, movies and the bombardment of advertising drive home the message that we should be happy. Even churches preach that being happy is the ultimate goal in life. It becomes the holy grail, the thing we hope for, that we seek with all our might. But being happy is closely linked to having a meaningful life. And many people have found that it is the meaning in their lives that make them happy, as Frankl said.

I have come to the conclusion that turning predicament into achievement is simply the only meaning there is.

This search for happiness may add meaning to your life – but why not rather search for meaning itself? Perhaps you cannot find happiness but find meaning instead and discover that meaning is the thing that brings you happiness. This is a hard lesson. In the concentration camp setting, inmates would just fail to get up and lie on their beds willing themselves to die. In the free (?) world, many people turn to drugs to fill their emptiness and lack of happiness. Those who cannot find meaning or happiness may eventually give up the search by committing suicide.

I have difficulty with those who maintain that everyone should be rich, healthy and happy. Even those who preach it from the Bible will have to explain why the Bible itself is proof that it is not the case. Think and grow rich, Napoleon Hill wrote, and thus he set the stage for the plethora of motivational speakers, writers and the like that followed, with the understanding that how you think, determines your life. This idea was not new, although it was received as such in the Western world. From a health perspective, Dr. Candace Pert and others have proved this to be scientifically true.

Does everything not hinge on definitions? What is happiness, what is health, what is joy? Different definitions of love are what drive couples apart who were initially attracted to each other. While the one might see love as doing things for the other (practical application) the other might see love from a romantic perspective and have the need to be wooed and romanced on an ongoing basis. The gulf between these definitions widens with each passing year, and if not addressed there would be only one way for a couple like this: one of them will be out the door eventually.

Likewise, the personal definition of happiness may mean one person may consider himself to be happy while another in similar conditions would not. Suffice to say that these concepts are personally adapted by each of us and that motivational speakers, preachers and the like hold to a universal definition that may be anathema to you as an individual.

The reality you accept in the waking state is known to you (mostly) from the impulses firing in your brain, while these impulses are linked to our senses. The sensation of touch has to be interpreted before it is classified as soft, scratchy, and so on. Thus the physical act of touching is not enough – the brain has to interpret what your fingers are experiencing. And there is no such a thing as your fingers experiencing touch, as separate or apart from, you yourself, your entire being, experiencing touching something soft.

Yet, Guy Claxton pointed out in The Wayward Mind, (Abacus 2005) that the brain is not a mechanism, but a system. He believes that the way our brains work does not necessarily match the way we think and talk.

And, with all the knowledge we have now on both the physiological, psychological and philosophical levels, we are nowhere near having enough knowledge to understand its functioning.

Frankl talks about the human being's capacity for self-detachment. I have experienced this first- hand. Firstly, the capacity to detach yourself from a situation (or surroundings). Those confined to hospital beds most certainly have to be able to do so. How otherwise would they remain human? Again Patch Adams comes to mind. He tried to remain connected to the humanness of the patients, going all the way against the norm prevalent in the medical system.

Then, Frankl also pointed out that there has to be a detachment from oneself. At certain times, I found that there was no other way to cope with what was happening than to detach myself from being myself. Or rather, being within the body that was failing me so profoundly. That the pain I was feeling was not me, even though I had come to define myself as a chronically ill person.

There is quite a difference between having a disease, and feeling as though you are the disease (being the disease). That point where being ill pervades your all, and defines who you are. I had a long hard fight out of this one.

Frankl called this capacity for self-detachment the basis of human freedom. Though we are not always conscious of the distinction between body and spirit, this is the point where your spirit becomes involved in what is going on in your body and chooses to react separately, as the need indicates. This can set you free from BEING the pain to being SOMEONE WITH PAIN.

Few people seek this detachment if they don't have to. It is of course prevalent in practices such as meditation and though I do not practice meditation I have become aware of how my spirit and physical body interact and the play between the two. I do not propound any theory or any practice in this regard. People find their own answers, based on how far and deep they are prepared to delve within themselves. Of course, on the furthest ends of this spectrum lie psychiatric disorders!

I don't think you should seek this detachment, I think it is something I had to come to terms with as a result of the pain and my movements being impaired. One can literally live in no other way than in your own mind. And your thought patterns do not extend into the unreachable, at the very start it did not reach very far at all. This is not surprising since just the act of getting out of bed had the status of reaching a mountain peak after hours of struggle. Over time though, thinking reaches out and becomes not just your link to reality, but your link to your own sanity.

"The conscious mind will enjoy no peace until it can rejoice in a fuller understanding of its own unconscious sources" said Lancelot Law Whyte, (referred to as the unconscious before Freud termed it the subconscious). When I read this I felt like rejoicing because it is utterly true of my own life experience.

Gay Claxton explained the web of meaning individuals weave for themselves as becoming their reality. The concepts and constructs learned as a child are the reality we build our lives on. Not surprisingly therefore, your thoughts (and your realities) depend on your culture. I was astounded at the vast difference in thinking between South Africans and Italians when I went to live in Italy for almost a year. Things I took for granted was anathema to them, and *vice versa*.

Claxton explained that the tales children are told at their mother's knee, become their implicit tales, which the culture accepts as common sense. These tales give people the code of thoughts that determine their conduct and which maintains the cohesion of their conduct. Think about it: the knight on his white horse coming to kiss the sleeping beauty awake, and them living happily ever after... we grow up with these archetypes created by the tales we were told. And we believe in little truths about life based on these tales.

"My world shows up to me pre-saturated with my own beliefs, memories and desires – yet how they got in there, I have no clue" according to Claxton.

Nietzsche said almost the same thing when he considered that the greater part of conscious thinking must still be counted among the instinctive activities. It is an instinctive, yet conscious move when I draw my hand back from a warm stove plate.

Thus, which of our conscious reactions are instinctive? Those, according to Claxton, we hold onto as intrinsic beliefs, otherwise known as common sense. Some might say there is nothing common about sense, but that might be a little too cynical a stance!

This could be why we so stubbornly believe that a doctor's prescription will heal a disease. It took me long enough to understand that doctors do not heal people but treat their symptoms. Perhaps they do effect healing, but that, I think, is limited to extreme, life-threatening situations. Long term, chronic diseases are treated – mostly with pharmaceutical means. Because we see it as an intrinsic belief.

Deepak Chopra points out that the body can reverse all processes it started, unlike the processes set in motion by taking a drug

Chapter Fifteen

Rising and running

Fifteen years of constant pain in my leg muscles left me with little hope beyond hobbling along. Then the pain started receding. It was hardly noticeable at first... it took me a few months before I realized that the pain was absent more often than it was present. Eventually I took it for granted that I no longer spent the nights rolling around in pain and the days clutching at my calf muscles in frustration. Now, more than 20 years down the line, I still have pain – sometimes. But it is manageable. It is neither constant, nor debilitating in its severity.

Another two years down the line (17 years after becoming ill), I decided to take up running. No, not jogging, *running*.

Some days, in fact most days, I ponder the miracle of being able to run. I know where I have been... the years of pain. The thousands of days I was less than a person, and more of a messy heap of muscle pain, dragging myself around in a sub-normal physical state.

myself? Perhaps even beyond the point of being able to participate? No, I am working up slowly to where I will prove not just to myself, but to everyone I have ever been in contact with, that the human spirit prevails over adversity – even if that is not its stated goal at the outset.

How does this feel, being able to jog – after the years of lying in a bed, curling with pain and unable to walk even a few hundred meters at a time? Does it even come to mind? It does so every time I put those running shoes on and get into my running gear. And the picture of that darkness pops into my mind when I feel my legs responding to my brain's instructions. Is it a miracle? I do believe it is.

The fact that I am running defies all the dire predictions of amputated feet and the like, which I have heard over the years, which, to my mind, is a miracle. It also defies the immovability to which I was subjected for months on end, and the muscular spasms I experienced for more than fifteen years.

I remember that very first time in a park that I jogged from tree to tree. I jogged no more than twenty paces – and felt buoyed by the fact that I was able to do so! Going back and forth a couple of times was enough for the first attempt.

Then I started doing sprints with a friend on the local soccer field. This too made it clear to me that I did have energy stores again. My muscles still had to catch up though. And while I was running from cone to cone I remembered my training days more than 40 years ago. Good memories came flooding back. The enjoyment of running around the track with my friends. Of doing cross country around the school. Those were the days.

And now, these are the days. I heard about Park Run from this friend and decided to take on a 5km distance. At the time that seemed near impossible. Imagine the feeling when finishing that distance. There I was, officially participating in an event with hundreds of others. What a thrill!

It was walk-jog-walk-jog all the way. But I made it to the end. And the one Park Run had me hooked. I realized that I could indeed do it. A few park runs later just making it to the end was not enough. I set my sights on going faster. After all, if you can do it in 34 minutes, you can do it in 33 also. This is the theory, right?

But I found that it was not a matter of doing it faster every time. Many things came into play. Various physical pains popped up.

The result of this pain was that I became more determined. Nothing was going to stop me. That it slowed me down, yes, sure, that was true. But give up? Stop running? No ways. One day may be a slow run, pushing through the pain. The next one may be better, faster, easier.

The first 30 runs I did were at the Voortrekker Monument in Pretoria. What a hill! I found out from weekly experience that the top of the hill was ever-elusive, just when you think you had rounded the last bend and would see the summit, you found yourself with another one.

That hill is a metaphor for life all right. I could have turned around at any moment and given up. I refused to do so. Not once have I ever failed to complete a race. In those early pre-fitness days it was walk/jog all the way to the top. But eventually it became jogging all the way – a triumph in itself.

After my 100th park run, I had an eight-week spate of PBs which made me think I was near invincible. Week after week I bettered my time, slicing minutes off my initial time, going from 34 min to just over 30minutes. When I plateaued the first time I had to learn acceptance. To keep trying despite my inability to run faster. Acceptance is not a singular exercise though. This is the same lesson I learned years ago when the illness struck me. One day at a time = one race at a time. And if it turns out to be disappointing, simply get up and do it again. Rise above the disappointment and keep trying.

Then early in 2019 I determined to participate in Masters Athletics. I was training for this and then came down with first bronchitis and then pneumonia – making training impossible. Since I missed the opportunity I formed the idea of running cross country. My daughter ran this for eight years – with me standing watching with varying levels of frustration. I wonder if she ever knew how much I wished that I could be running, too?

Initially the plan was for the two of us to run together. Yet when the day arrived she was no longer running. I supposed I could have given up on the idea then. But I am a rather determined person. Once I have committed myself, I see things through. Thus there I was, all by myself, in the starting line at the first event of the season. Very early on in the race we hit zig-zags. Just there my left knee made itself felt. It did not like the movement at all. Zigzags are not sharp corners. They force a momentary stop and direction change. This is not a fluid movement, particularly not to the uninitiated.

That first cross country run was utter hell. I did not enjoy it. I quite vocally let it be known that I now understood why my daughter never liked it.

"Why do people even run it?" I kept asking myself. Yet, next league run, there I was again at the starting line. This one was far worse! By now my knee was niggling all the way through running. And this run had uphills that seemed innocuous at first, but turned out to be vicious. While running I commented to those watching us suffer that this was murder for oldies.

The distance for my age group is 4km and I started the season on just over 26 minutes. Of course this was nothing to brag about… time-wise. But the fact that I had niggling pain, also sciatica that stuck to me like my best friend, made every run a challenge. It was no fun!

Our league rules demand that one runs at least three races prior to champs. This I did. And found that despite the physical problems, I managed to cut my time every week. By the time provincial champs came around, I completed that race in just over 24 minutes.

Early September there we were on a bitterly cold morning, at the murderous course once again, for national championships. I was THRILLED TO RUN that morning. And never had I enjoyed anything more than that day. Here I was, 38 years after having last trained or participated in an official race, running South African championships.

That race was a triumph on all counts. I was with thousands of others participating on the national level – against the best. Me! Me without my ME....!

I can feel the sun, the wind against my face, and I can run. Thank you, Lord.

Famous? No. Beautiful? No. Successful? No. not in the worldly sense the word implies. But alive and kicking... yes. On that dark morning I woke up dead. But fought myself back to a running life.

[For the record I bettered my time at the national championships with another 1:05 seconds. I am training every day for the upcoming season.]